FAT BOMBS

The Complete Keto Fat Bombs Cookbook

160 Sweet and Savory Keto Snacks Recipes for Healthy Eating to Lose Weight Fast

---

2 Manuscripts in 1 Book

Adele Baker

This book is dedicated to my little daughter, my inspiration and my soul

---

Disclaimer

Images from shutterstock.com

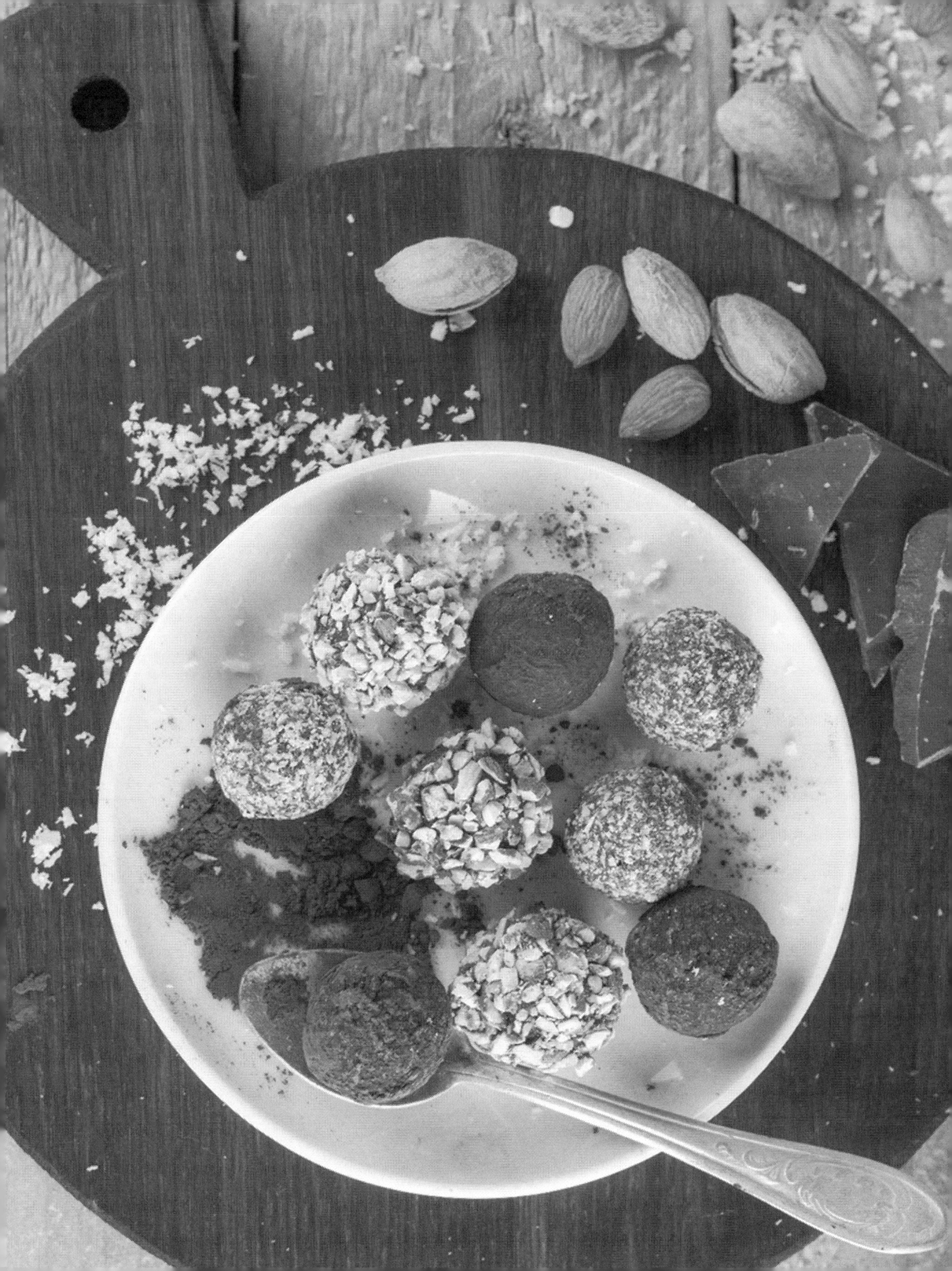

Your Gift

Sign up to my newsletter for free Kindle books.

By joining my newsletter, you will be notified when my books are free on Amazon, so you can download them and not have to pay!

You will also be notified when I release a new book and be able to buy it for a reduced price.

Now you will get for free **TOP recipes for any occasion from the best-selling author Adele Baker**

All files will be delivered to your inbox (in PDF format) and can be read on your laptop, phone, or tablet.

Just click the link below to signup and receive your free book:

http://www.adelebaker.com/promo/recipesfortwo/from/fatbombs

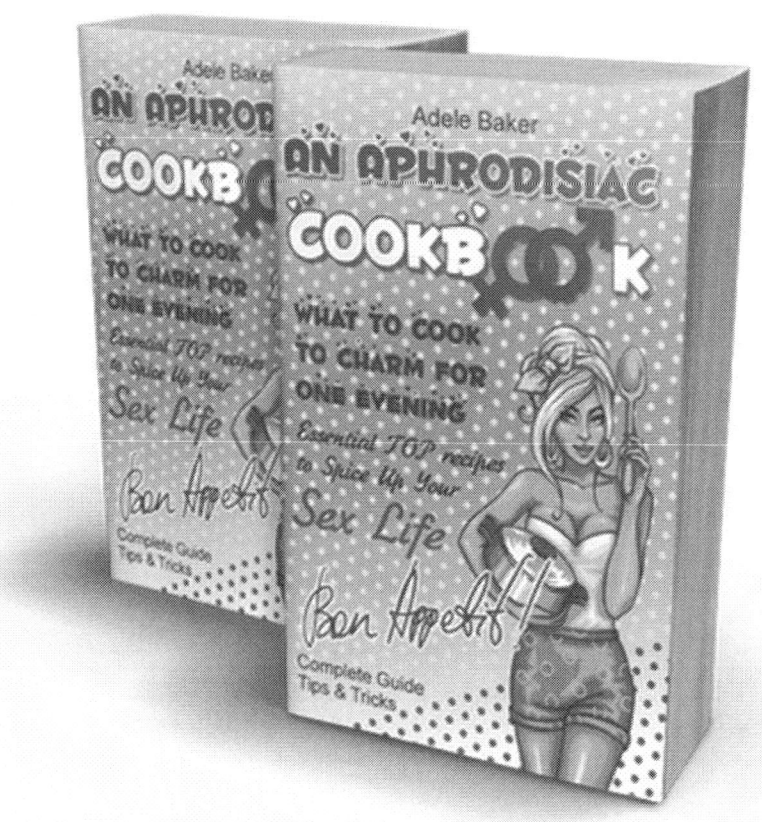

I know you will love this gift!

Thanks, and enjoy!

CONTENTS

SWEET FAT BOMBS 138

Keto Fat Bombs

70 Sweet & Savory Recipes for Ketogenic, Paleo & Low-Carb Diets

Adele Baker

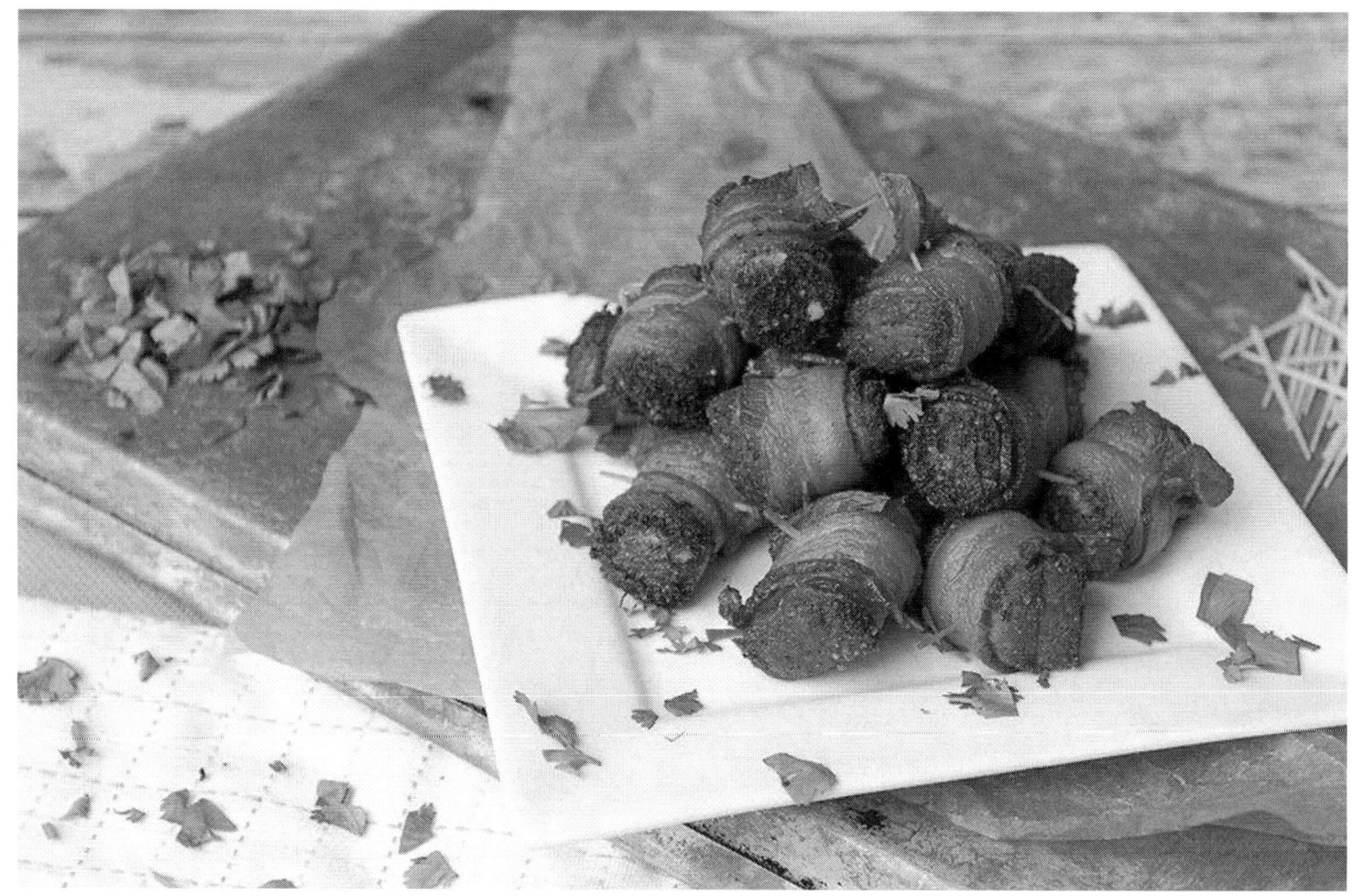

INTRODUCTION

What do you imagine when you hear the phrase "fat bomb"? Most likely it frightens you, especially if you are struggling with excess weight or just trying to keep fit. But do not be afraid, some fats can even be beneficial (e.g., coconut cream, coconut butter, coconut oil, cream cheese). That's the main point when including fat bombs in your ketogenic (keto) meal plan.

I strongly believe that if you are on a keto diet, you should eat all the right meals and do all possible to make this diet beneficial. If you're following your macronutrients (macros) and eating them diligently, then you're doing an excellent job. But still some problems may exist with getting the proper amounts of macros, especially fats, and here fat bombs come into play! These bite-sized snacks are loaded down with fat, containing a good portion of the recommended daily amount in just one serving.

Keto dieters use a wide variety of fat bomb recipes. Most of them include a combination of coconut flakes, vanilla, cacao powder, dark chocolate, cinnamon, peanut butter, almond butter, cocoa butter, cheese, coconut cream, bacon bits and more. The keto fat bombs can be savory or sweet. There are no strict rules about making them,! It is incredibly easy. All you need to do is combine your ingredients, and then form this mixture into small balls that are easy to handle and eat or use a cute mold to give your fat bombs a unique shape.

Want to make some of these for yourself? This book will provide you with a complete guide to keto fat bombs, giving all necessary information and basic principles for successful incorporation of fat bombs into your dietary plan. Seventy delicious recipes of sweet and savory fat bombs are included. Enjoy foods that are tasty and beneficial at the same time!

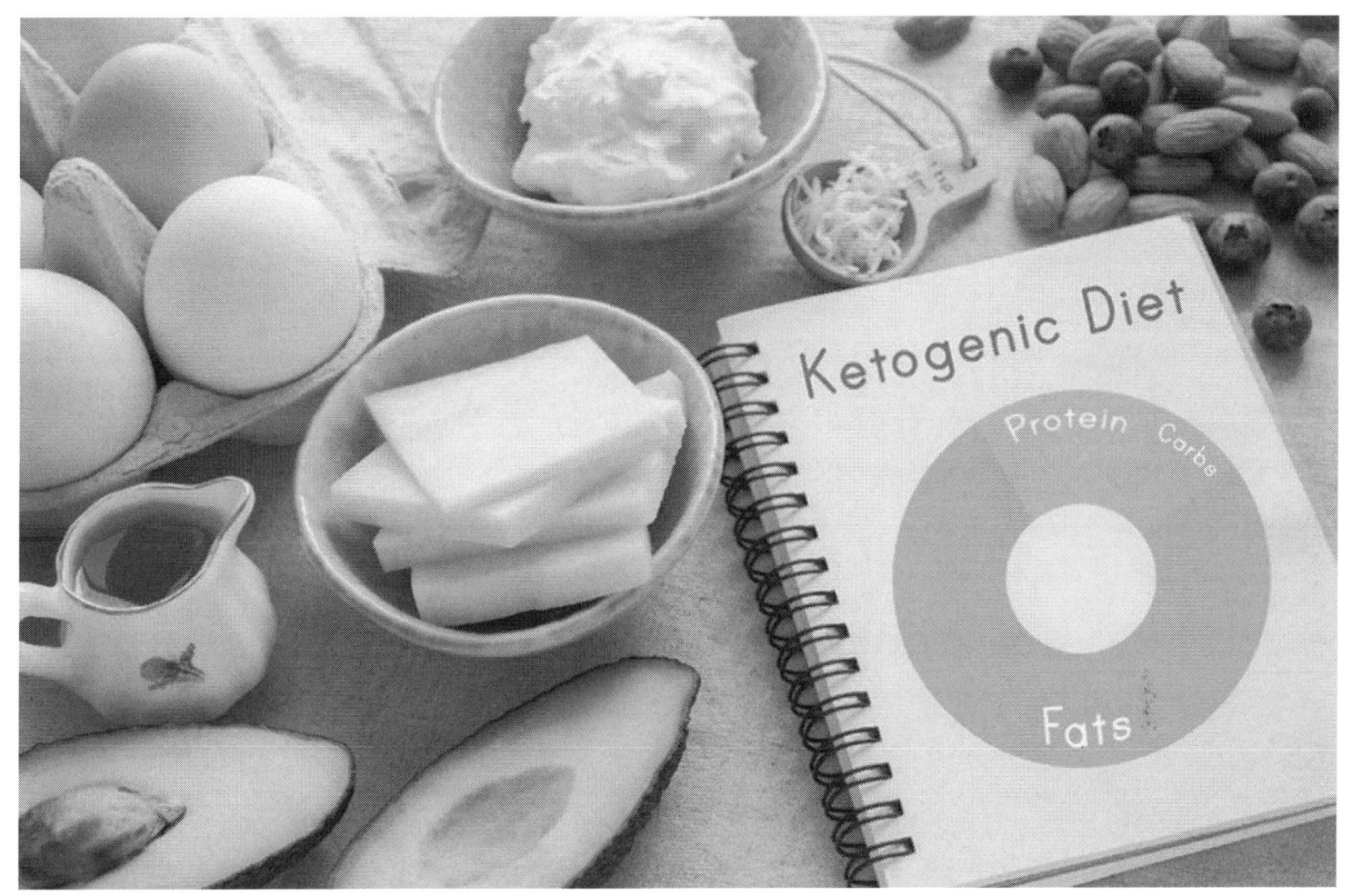

What is Keto?

The ketogenic diet is low carbohydrate (carb), high fat and moderate protein diet that puts the body into a metabolic state called ketosis. In other words, the diet involves radically reducing carbohydrate intake and substituting it with fat.

When your foods are high in carbs your body will produce glucose and insulin:

- Glucose is an energy source that is the easiest for our bodies to convert into energy and use. Thus it will be chosen over any other energy source.
- Insulin is a hormone that processes the glucose so that your bloodstream can distribute it around your body.

Since glucose is the main form of energy, fats are not used and are, therefore, stored. Typically on a normal, higher carbohydrate diet, the body will use glucose as its primary energy source. But due to the incredible adaptive abilities of our bodies, we can induce it into a state known as ketosis by lowering the intake of carbs.

Ketosis is a natural process the body uses to help us survive when food intake is low. During this state, chemicals called ketones are produced. This process is started not by a lack of calories, but by a lack of carbohydrates.

Types of Keto Diet

- Standard ketogenic diet (SKD): This is a very low-carb, moderate-protein and high-fat diet. It typically includes 75% fat, 20% protein and only 5% carbs

- Cyclical ketogenic diet (CKD): This diet involves periods of higher-carb "refeeds"; for example, 5 ketogenic days followed by 2 high-carb days
- Targeted ketogenic diet (TKD): This diet involves adding carbs around physical workouts
- High-protein ketogenic diet: This has features in common with a standard ketogenic diet, but contains more protein. It contains 60% fat, 35% protein and 5% carbs

Benefits of a Ketogenic Diet

✓ **Weight Loss**

Using fats as an energy source, the ketogenic diet promotes considerable weight loss. Being on a keto diet, your insulin levels fall greatly which actually turns your body into a fat burning machine. Furthermore, the ketogenic diet has proved to have better results then low-fat and high-carb diets.

✓ **Control Blood Sugar**

The keto diet is thought to decrease blood sugar levels mainly because of the types of foods you consume. Studies even reveal that the ketogenic dietary pattern is a more effective way to prevent diabetes than low-calorie diets. You need to consider this diet if you are pre-diabetic or have type 2 diabetes. Many people have success managing their blood sugar on the keto diet.

✓ **Mental Focus**

By adopting the ketogenic diet, many people are able to increase their mental performance. That's because ketones are a great source of fuel for the brain. By lowering carb intake, you prevent big spikes in blood sugar. These factors can have a positive effect on focus and concentration. Another factor is that an increased intake of fatty acids can have some benefits on our brain's function.

✓ **Increased Energy & Normalized Hunger**

Fat has been shown to be the most effective fuel to burn as an energy source. By giving your body a better and more reliable fuel, you will be more energetic during the day. Moreover, fat is naturally more satisfying food, so we feel full for a longer time.

What to Eat and What to Avoid on the Keto Diet

You should base most of your meals around these foods:

Meat & Seafood

- Alligator
- Bacon
- Bear
- Beef
- Bison
- Bison Jerky
- Bison Ribeye
- Bison Sirloin
- Bison Steaks
- Boar
- Chicken Breast
- Chicken Leg
- Chicken Thigh
- Chicken Wings
- Chuck Steak
- Clams
- Crab
- Duck
- Eggs (chicken, duck, goose)
- Elk
- Emu
- Goat
- Goose
- Ground Beef
- Ground lamb
- Ham
- Hot dogs
- Kangaroo
- Kielbasa
- Lamb Chops
- Lamb Rack
- Lobster
- Mussels
- New York Steak
- Ostrich
- Oysters
- Pheasant
- Pork
- Pork Chops
- Poultry
- Quail
- Rabbit

- Rattlesnake
- Reindeer
- Salmon
- Sausage
- Scallop
- Shrimp
- Spam
- Steak
- Trout
- Turkey
- Turtle
- Veal
- Venison Steaks

Dairy

- Blue Cheese
- Brie
- Butter
- Cheddar Cheese
- Colby Jack Cheese
- Cottage Cheese
- Cream Cheese
- Feta Cheese
- Goat Cheese
- Gouda
- Heavy Whipping Cream
- Mozzarella Cheese
- Parmesan Cheese
- Provolone Cheese
- Ricotta
- Sour Cream
- Swiss Cheese
- Unsweetened Greek Yogurt
- Unsweetened Plain Yogurt

Vegetables

- Alfalfa Sprouts
- Artichoke
- Arugula
- Asparagus
- Avocado

- Banana Peppers
- Beet Greens
- Bok Choy
- Broccoli
- Broccoli Rabe (Rapini)
- Brussels Sprouts
- Butterhead Lettuce
- Cabbage
- Cauliflower
- Celery
- Chard
- Chayote
- Chicory Greens
- Collard Greens
- Cucumber
- Eggplant
- Endive
- Escarole
- Green Beans
- Iceberg Lettuce
- Jalapeño Pepper
- Jicama
- Kohlrabi
- Mung Bean
- Mushroom
- Mustard Greens
- Nori
- Okra
- Potato
- Radish
- Red Tomatoes
- Romaine
- Rutabaga
- Spaghetti Squash
- Spinach
- Summer Squash
- Tomatillo
- Turnip
- Water Spinach
- Yellow Tomatoes
- Zucchini

Berries

- Strawberries
- Blueberries
- Raspberries
- Cranberries
- Mulberries

Leafy Greens

- Spinach
- Kale

Nuts and seeds

- Macadamias
- Walnuts
- Sunflower
- Seeds

Sweeteners

- Stevia
- Erythritol
- Monk Fruit
- Xylitol

Fats & Oils

- Animal Fats
- Avocado Oil
- Butter
- Cocoa Butter
- Coconut Oil
- Flaxseed Oil
- Ghee (Clarified Butter)
- Hemp Oil
- Lard
- Macadamia Oil
- Mayonnaise
- Olive Oil
- Palm Oil
- Peanut Oil
- Pumpkin Seed Oil
- Red Palm Oil
- Sesame Oil
- Tallow
- Tea Seed Oil
- Walnut Oil

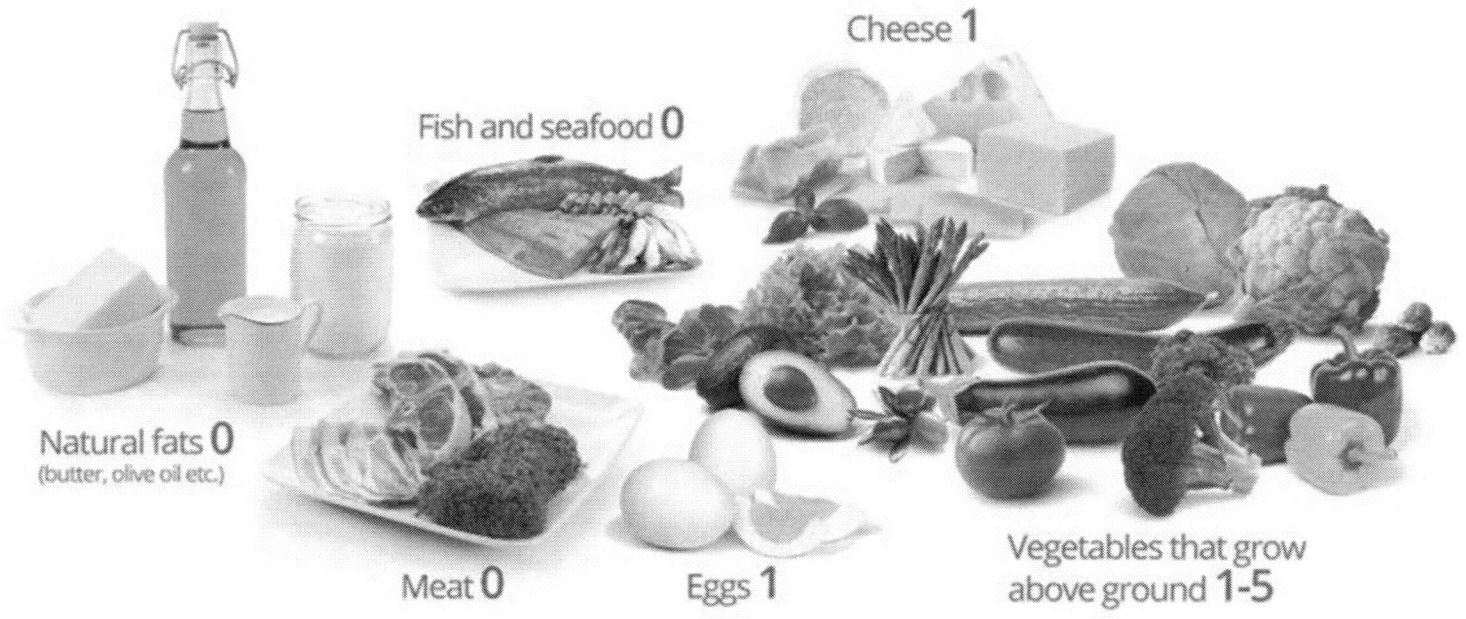

Cheese 1

Fish and seafood 0

Natural fats 0
(butter, olive oil etc.)

Meat 0

Eggs 1

Vegetables that grow
above ground 1-5

Foods that you should reduce on a Ketogenic Diet

Grains

- Wheat
- Corn
- Rice
- Cereal
- Rye
- Oats
- Barley

- Millet
- Bulgur
- Sorghum
- Amaranth
- Buckwheat
- Quinoa

Sugar

- Honey
- Agave
- Maple syrup

Fruit

- Apples
- Bananas
- Oranges and Other Citrus

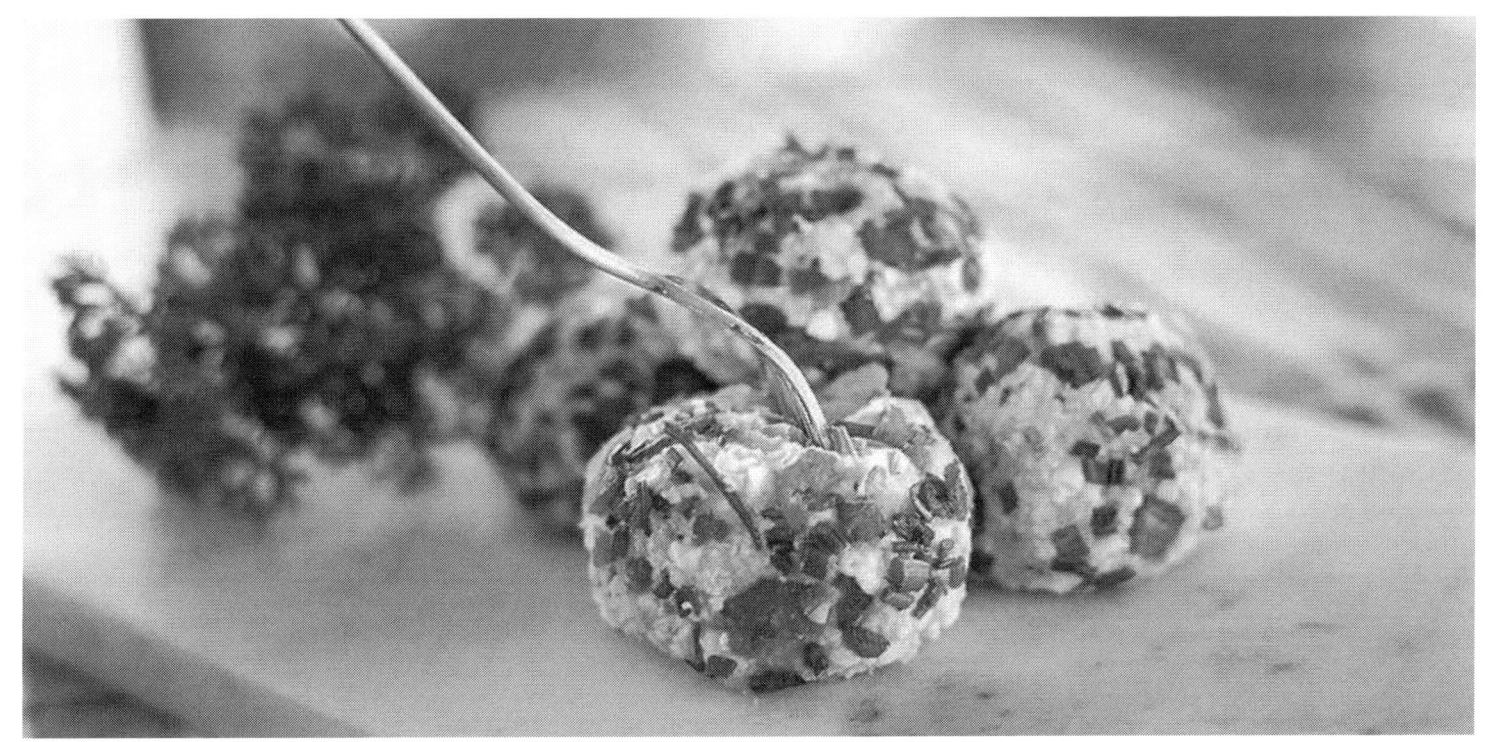

What are Fat Bombs?

When searching for different keto recipes, you will surely come across something called a "fat bomb". When hearing this term, you actually imagine greasy junk food like a large bowl of ice cream topped with syrup, a candy bar, or a burger. But when talking about keto fat bombs, the meaning is absolutely different. This is a small snack which is high in fat and low in protein and carbohydrates—the ideal snack if you're on a low carb diet. Giving you an easy way to eat healthy fats, fat bombs help provide your body with 70-75% of the daily rate for fats. There exists a great variety of recipes that you can use to make yourself a snack with incredible flavor—and that's while being on a diet.

Fat bombs are especially useful on those days when, as much as you eat, you just can't seem to get your necessary fat rate. This often happens during busy days when you have no time to eat much more than a salad, or when you can't do much cooking for one reason or another. For such situations, fat bombs are just perfect because they are easy to make and to store, and always ready to go.

Facts about keto fat bombs so you can better understand them:

1. Ketogenic fat bombs are usually small

Being so high in fat, fat bombs cannot be eaten in big portions, so they usually have the size of small balls or mini-muffins. The most convenient way to make them is to use a muffin pan with liners and to pour the mixture into the pan This way your hands won't get dirty while making the mixture. You can easily take several bombs with you to eat on your way to work or to the gym.

2. Fat bombs can be savory or sweet

We can divide fat bombs into two groups: sweet and savory. The first one tends to be sweet (usually because of sweeteners like stevia). Such sweeteners are low calorie (and zero carbs) and don't cause harm to your health, unlike those sugar alcohols that some low-carb treats contain. You can use your own low-carb sweetener of choice for sweet keto fat bombs. Savory fat bombs are mainly considered ones made with such ingredients as bacon, avocado, etc.

3. Fat bombs contain lots of healthy fats

As was already mentioned, fat bombs contain lots of fat. Most ketogenic fat bombs contain mainly coconut oil or coconut butter as an ingredient. Besides its nutritional value, coconut oil is also helpfpful for the recipe since it solidifies when refrigerated, making these fat bombs a lot less messy to eat.

4. Fat bombs should be stored refrigerated

The best way to store the fat bombs is to refrigerate then because fat is often liquid at room temperature. They can be kept for 1-2 weeks in the fridge in an airtight container. You can also freeze them, although it can be a nuisance because you have to thaw them first before eating as they can get very hard.

5. Fat bombs often also contain nuts and seeds

Try not to eat too many nuts and seeds on a ketogenic diet since some nuts and seeds are actually quite rich in carbs. Furthermore, the fats in nuts and seeds can become easily oxidized if the recipe requires them to be heated.

Here are some tips on how to consume fat bombs on the keto diet:

- Use fat bombs as a quick hit of energy when you don't have time to cook.
- Use them as pre- or post-workout snacks instead of "regular" snacks that are high in carbs.
- Consume fat bombs to boast your fat intake to meet the macronutrient targets. Almost 80 percent of the calories in the recipes in this cookbook come from fats.

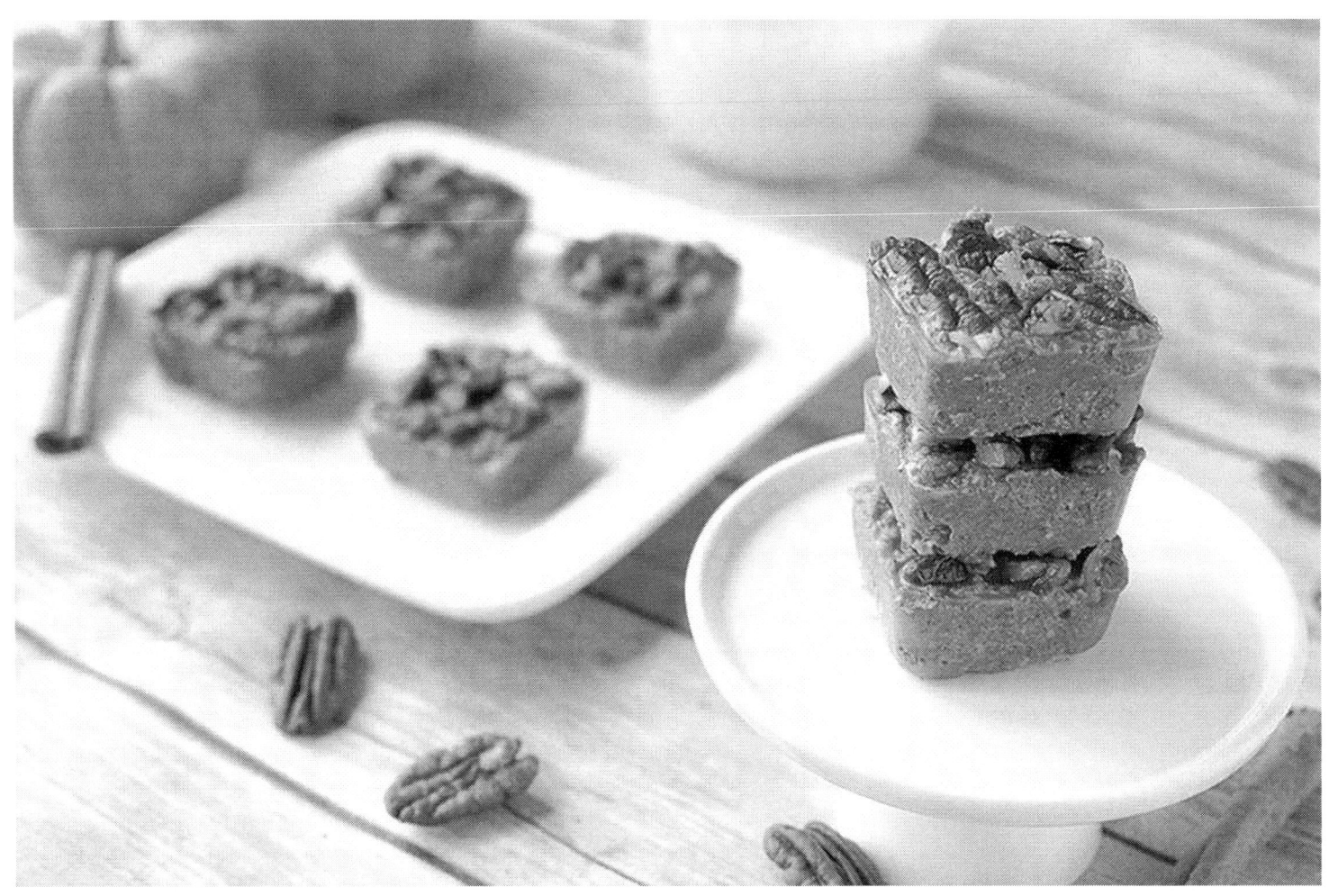

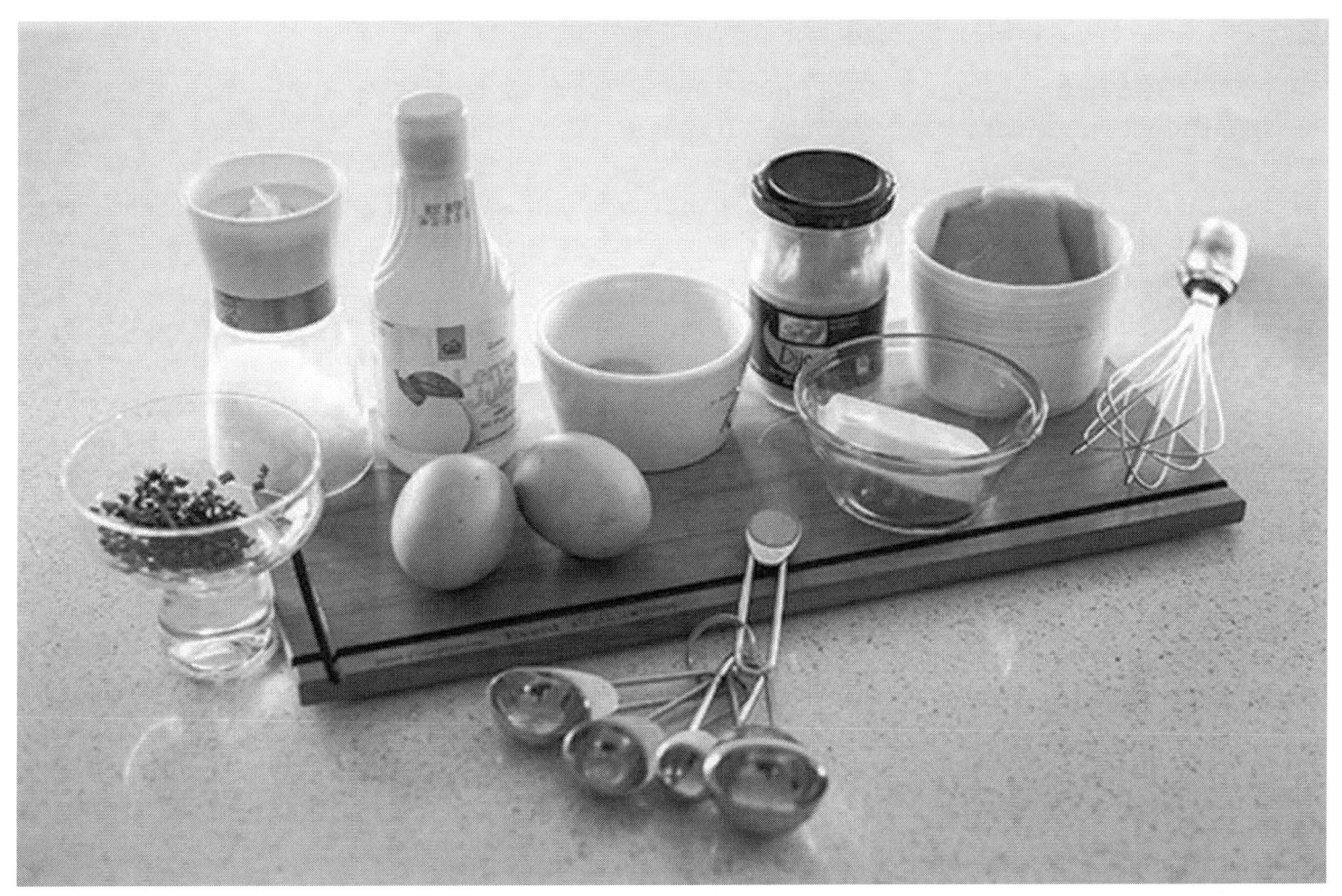

How to Make Fat Bombs

3 basic ingredients are in every fat bomb recipe:

1. Healthy Fats:

- cacao butter
- coconut butter
- almond butter
- coconut oil
- coconut milk
- coconut cream (solid part of a refrigerated can of coconut milk)
- ghee (mostly lactose and casein free, especially if you get cultured ghee, so it doesn't present the same problems as other dairy products)
- butter (ok if you're not sensitive to dairy)
- bacon fat
- avocado oil

2. Flavoring:

- sugar-free vanilla extract
- 100% dark chocolate
- cacao powder
- salt
- peppermint extract
- spices

3. Texture:

- cacao nibs
- almonds
- pecans
- walnuts
- chia seeds
- bacon bits (choose sugar-free)
- shredded coconut

The main steps in cooking fat bombs:

- **STEP 1:** Combine all the needed ingredients in a mixing bowl, a food processor or a blender, depending on the consistency you need. If using solid fat (e.g., coconut oil), melt it slightly in the microwave.
- **STEP 2:** To make small balls, pour the mixture into muffin cups or into a baking pan, or just use your hands to form the needed shape.
- **STEP 3:** Refrigerate (or freeze) for several hours for the mixture to become solid. Cut into pieces if using a baking pan.

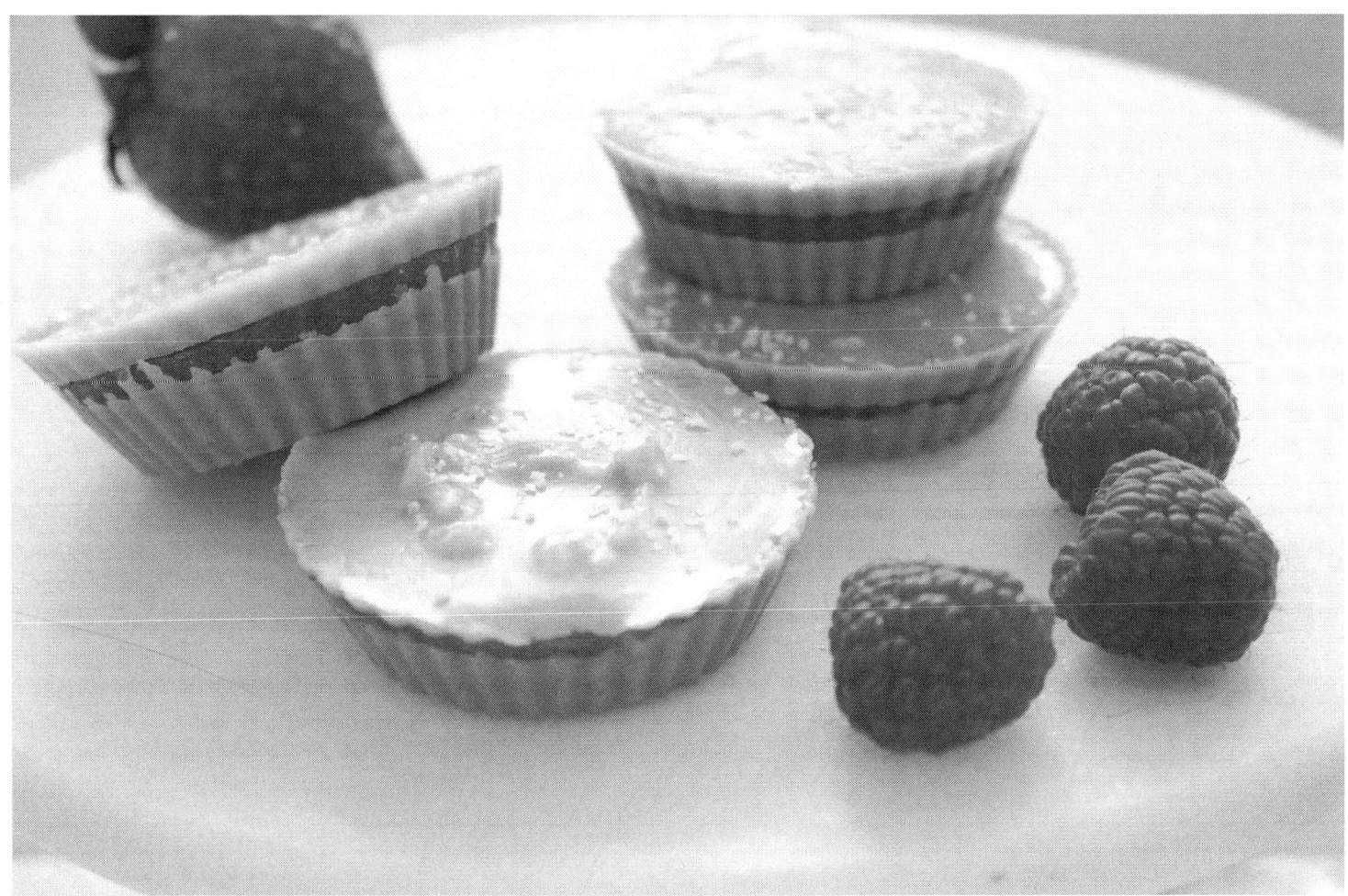

SAVORY FAT BOMBS

Bacon & Egg Fat Bombs

Prep time: 10 min (+ 30 min)

Cooking time: 15 min

Servings: 6

Nutrients per serving:

Total Carbs – 0.2 g

Net Carbs – 0.2 g

Fat –18.4 g

Protein – 5 g

Calories – 185

Ingredients:

- 2 large eggs, hard-boiled, cut into quarters
- ¼ cup butter
- 2 tbsp mayonnaise
- 4 large slices bacon
- Salt, pepper to taste

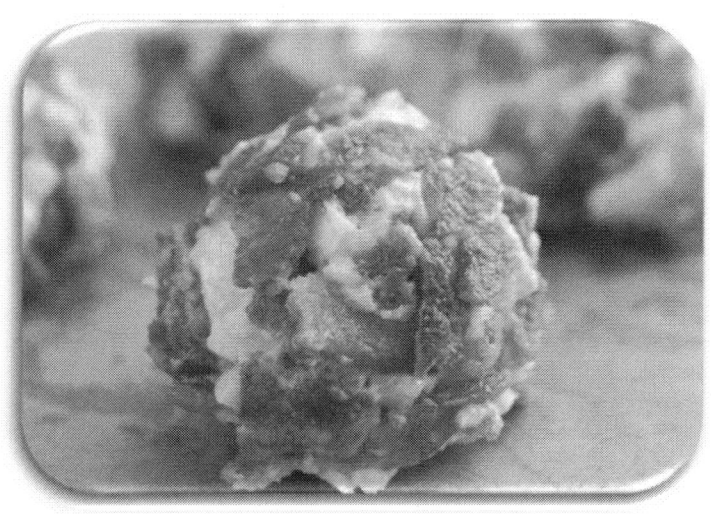

Instructions:

1. Preheat the oven to 375 °F.
2. Cook the bacon strips on a baking tray for 15 minutes. Reserve the grease.
3. Cut the butter into pieces and add the quartered eggs. Mash with a fork to mix.
4. Add the remaining ingredients except for the bacon and mix. Pour in the bacon grease. Mix well. Refrigerate for 20-30 minutes.
5. Crumble the bacon. Create 6 balls from egg mixture and roll each ball in the bacon crumbles.
6. Serve.

Bacon & Guacamole Fat Bombs

Prep time: 10 min (+ 30 min)

Cooking time: 15 min

Servings: 6

Nutrients per serving:

Total Carbs – 2.7 g

Fiber – 1.3 g

Net Carbs – 1.4 g

Fat –15.2 g

Protein – 3.4 g

Calories – 156

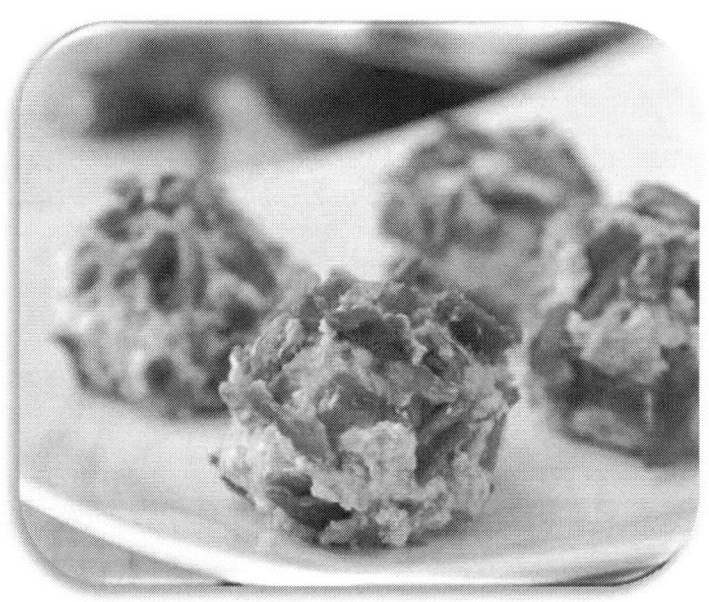

Ingredients:

- ½ avocado, peeled, halved
- ¼ cup butter
- 2 cloves garlic, crushed
- 1 chili pepper, chopped
- 2 tbsp cilantro, chopped
- 1 tbsp lime juice
- ½ onion, diced
- 4 slices bacon
- Salt, pepper to taste

Instructions:

1. Preheat the oven to 375°F.
2. Cook the bacon strips on a baking tray for 15 minutes. Reserve the grease.
3. Combine the first six ingredients. Season with salt, pepper to taste and mix.
4. Add the onion and the bacon grease and mix. Refrigerate for 20-30 minutes.
5. Crumble the bacon. Create 6 balls from the mixture. Roll each ball in the bacon crumbles.
6. Serve.

Mediterranean Fat Bombs

Prep time: 10 min (+30 min)

Cooking time: 0 min

Servings: 5

Nutrients per serving:

Total Carbs – 2 g

Fiber – 0.3 g

Net Carbs – 1.7 g

Fat –17.1 g

Protein – 3.7 g

Calories – 164

Ingredients:

- ½ cup full-fat cream cheese
- ¼ cup butter
- 2 tsp dried herbs
- 4 sun-dried tomatoes, chopped
- 4 kalamata olives, chopped
- 2 cloves garlic, crushed
- 5 tbsp Parmesan cheese, grated
- Salt, pepper to taste

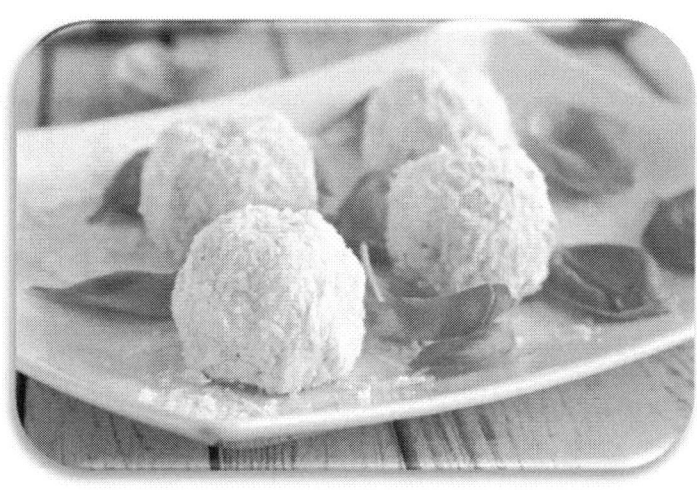

Instructions:

1. Combine butter with the cream cheese. Mash with a fork to mix.
2. Mix in remaining ingredients except for the Parmesan cheese. Refrigerate 30 minutes.
3. Create 5 balls out of the cheese mixture. Cover each ball with the grated parmesan cheese.
4. Serve or store in a container in the refrigerator

Pizza Fat Bombs

Prep time: 20 min

Cooking time: 0 min

Servings: 6

Nutrients per serving:

Total Carbs – 2 g

Net Carbs – 1.69 g

Fat – 9.62 g

Protein – 2.3 g

Calories – 101.3

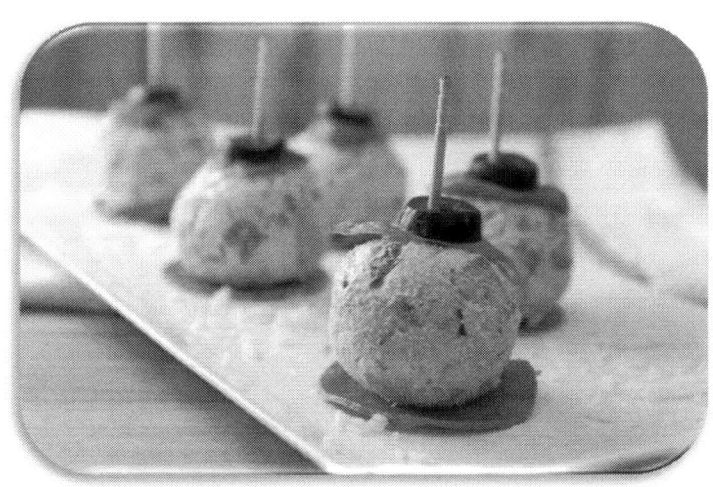

Ingredients:

- 4 oz cream cheese
- 14 slices pepperoni
- 8 pitted black olives
- 2 tbsp sun-dried tomato pesto
- 2 tbsp chopped fresh basil
- Salt, pepper to taste

Instructions:

1. Chop pepperoni and olives into small pieces.
2. Combine cream cheese, basil, and tomato pesto.
3. Mix the olives and pepperoni with the cream cheese.
4. Form into balls. Serve.

Jalapeño Pepper Fat Bombs

Prep time: 20 min

Cooking time: 5 min

Servings: 6

Nutrients per serving:

Total Carbs – 2.36 g

Net Carbs – 2.13 g

Fat –13.3 g

Protein – 4.77 g

Calories – 147

Ingredients:

- 3 oz cream cheese
- 3 slices bacon
- 1 jalapeño pepper, seeded
- ½ tsp parsley, dried
- ¼ tsp onion powder
- ¼ tsp garlic powder
- Salt, pepper to taste

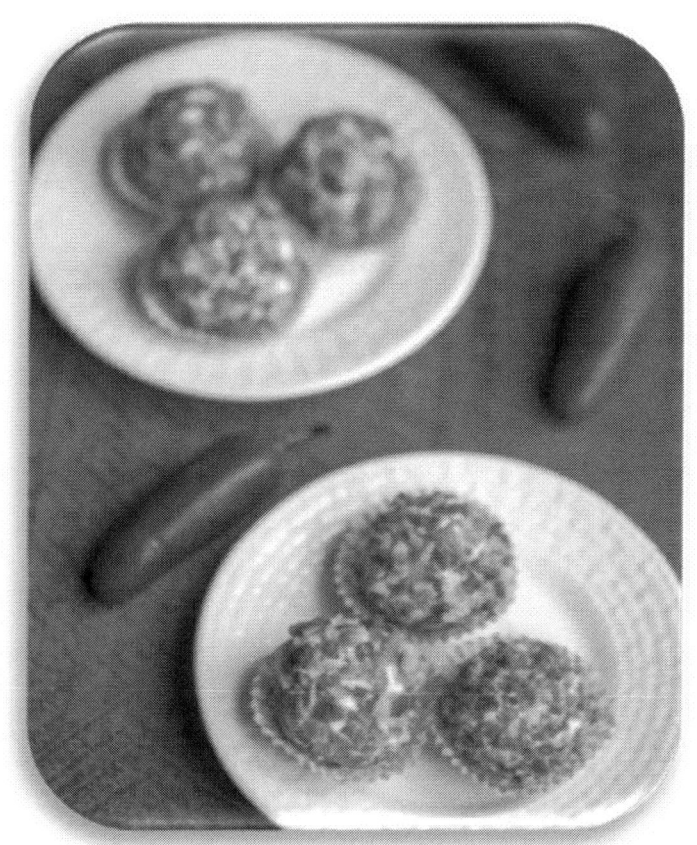

Instructions:

1. Fry bacon slices for 5 minutes, then place them on paper towels. Save bacon grease.
2. Chop the jalapeño pepper. Mix together with cream cheese, bacon fat, and spices.
3. Make balls out of cream cheese mixture and roll them in the crumbled bacon. Serve or store refrigerated in a container.

Waldorf Salad Fat Bombs

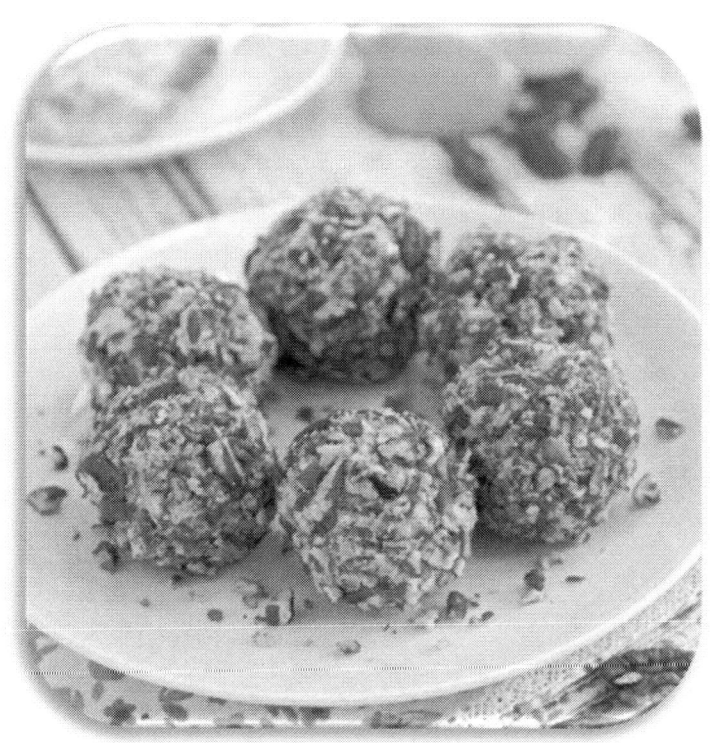

Prep time: 15 min (+ 30 min)

Cooking time: 0 min

Servings: 24

Nutrients per serving:

Total Carbs – 4 g

Net Carbs – 2.5 g

Fat – 19.3 g

Protein – 4.5 g

Calories – 193

Ingredients:

- 3 oz full-fat cream cheese
- 2 tbsp unsalted butter
- ½ cup blue cheese, crumbled
- ½ green apple, peeled, diced
- ¼ tsp garlic powder
- ¼ tsp onion powder
- 2 tbsp chives, chopped
- 2/3 cup pecans, chopped
- Salt, pepper to taste

Instructions:

1. Mash together the cream cheese and butter.
2. Add the remaining ingredients except for pecans. Mix well. Refrigerate 30 minutes.
3. Make 6 balls out of the mixture. Roll the balls in the chopped pecans. Serve.

Zucchini Fat Bombs

Prep time: 5 min (+ 2 hr)

Cooking time: 30 min

Servings: 12

Nutrients per serving:

Total Carbs – 2.5 g

Net Carbs – 0.48 g

Fat –13.65 g

Protein – 2 g

Calories – 157

Ingredients:

- 1 zucchini
- 3.5 oz cream cheese
- 1 oz Cheddar cheese
- 1 oz Parmesan cheese
- 1.5 oz unsalted butter
- Salt to taste

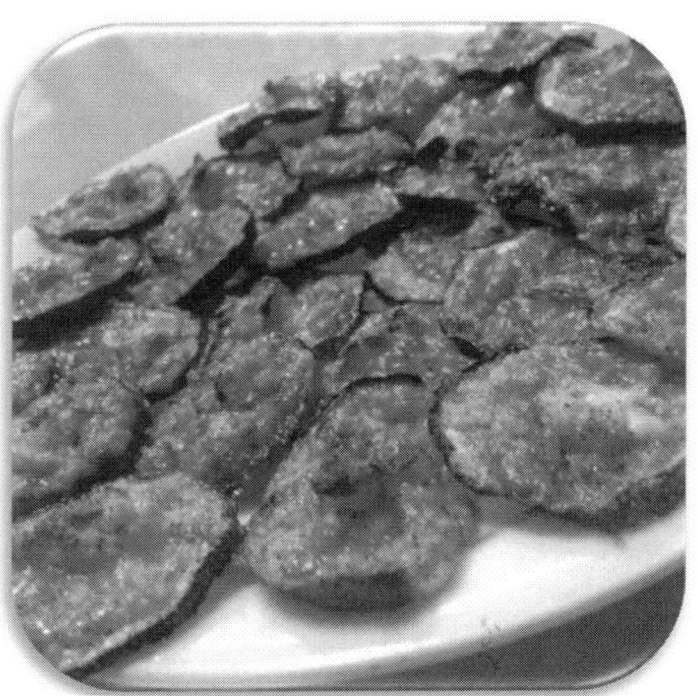

Instructions:

1. Slice zucchini. In a nonstick pan lay slices of zucchini in rows—each with a bit of butter on top and bottom.
2. Add cream cheese and Cheddar in the center of each slice, and then sprinkle Parmesan cheese all over. Season with salt.
3. Heat the oven to 220°F. Cook for 30 minutes or until golden. Let cool and serve.

Broiled Bacon Wraps with Dates

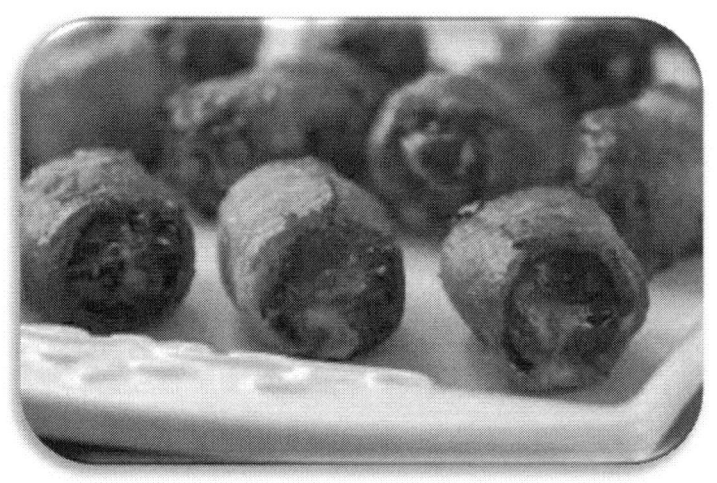

Prep time: 40 minutes

Cooking time: 15 minutes

Servings: 6

Nutrition facts per serving:

Total carbs – 5 g

Protein – 19 g

Total fat – 10 g

Calories – 203

Ingredients:

- 8 oz dates, pitted, slit
- 1 lb bacon, sliced

Instructions:

1. Wrap each date with ½ slice bacon and secure with a toothpick.
2. Arrange the bacon wraps on a baking tray and bake at 425°F for 15-18 minutes.

Smoked Mackerel Pâté Fat Bombs

Prep time: 10 min (+ 30 min)

Cooking time: 0 min

Servings: 6

Nutrients per serving:

Total Carbs – 0.8 g

Net Carbs – 0.7 g

Fat – 17.3 g

Protein – 4.9 g

Calories – 161

Ingredients:

- 3.5 oz full-fat cream cheese
- ¼ cup unsalted butter
- 1 mackerel fillet, smoked
- 1 tbsp lime juice
- 2 tbsp fresh chives, chopped
- 6 cucumber slices

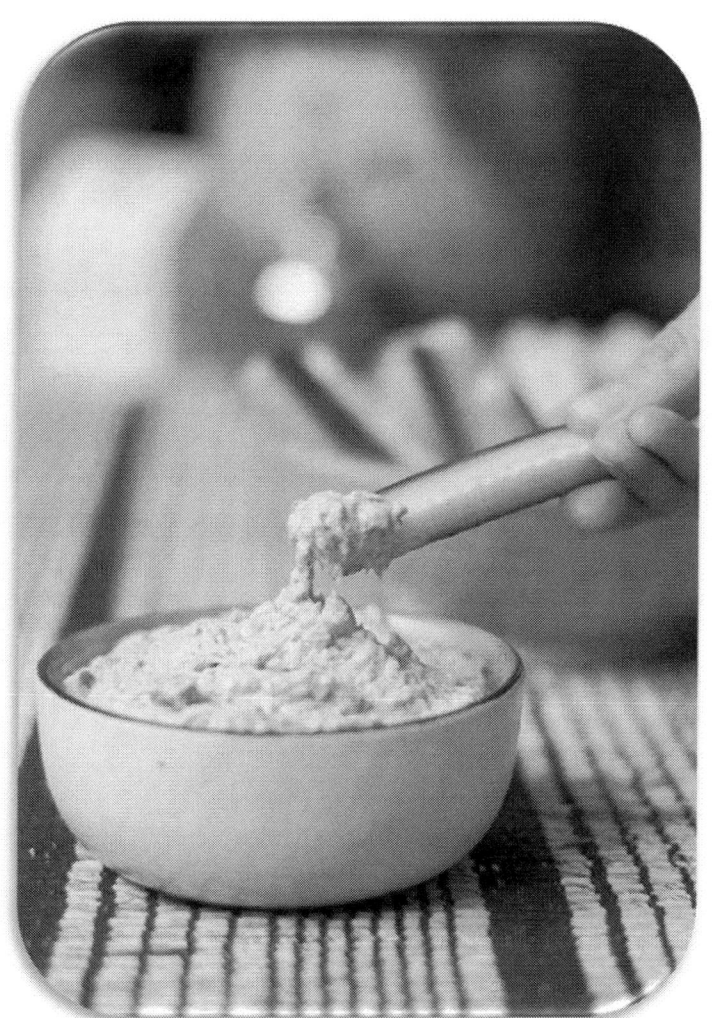

Instructions:

1. In a food processor, blend first four ingredients.
2. In a bowl, combine the mixture with the chives, and mix with a spoon. Refrigerate for 30 minutes.
3. Serve as a dip with cucumber slices or store in an airtight container in the fridge for up to a week.

Smoked Salmon Canapés

Prep time: 5 minutes

Cooking time: none

Servings: 4

Nutrients per serving:

Total Carbs – 5 g

Fat – 2.4 g

Protein – 2.6 g

Calories – 51

Ingredients:

- 6 oz smoked salmon, cut into small squares
- 1 avocado, halved, pitted
- 1 cucumber, sliced in rounds
- 10 black olives, chopped
- 1 tsp lemon juice
- 1 sprig fresh dill

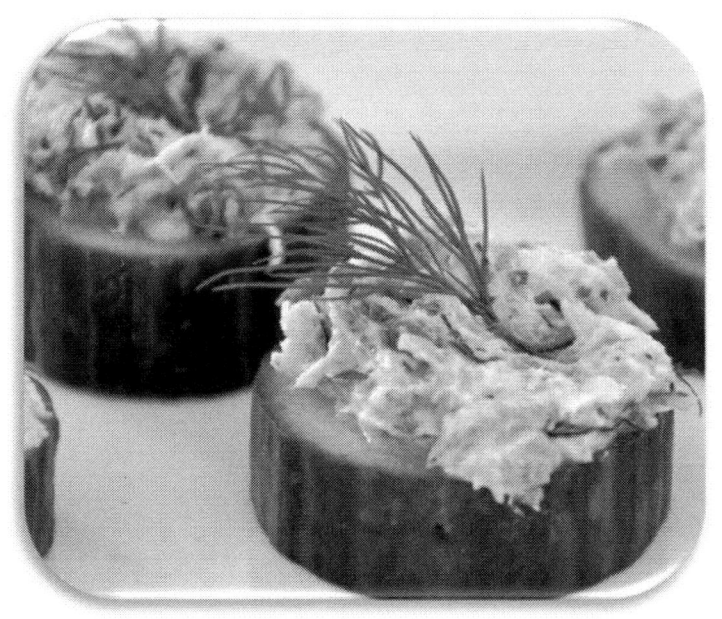

Instructions:

1. Mash avocado with lemon juice.
2. Combine smoked salmon and olives with avocado.
3. Spread a thin layer of avocado salmon mixture on a cucumber slice.
4. Decorate with fresh dill.

Bacon and Pâté Fat Bombs

Prep time: 20 min (+ 30 min)

Cooking time: 35 min

Servings: 6

Nutrients per serving:

Total Carbs –.,4 g

Net Carbs – 1.2 g

Fat –19.8 g

Protein – 7 g

Calories – 213

Ingredients:

- 4 large bacon slices
- 1/3 cup unsalted butter, divided
- 5.5 oz chicken livers, diced
- ½ onion, diced
- 2 garlic cloves, chopped
- 1 tbsp fresh sage, chopped
- Salt, pepper to taste

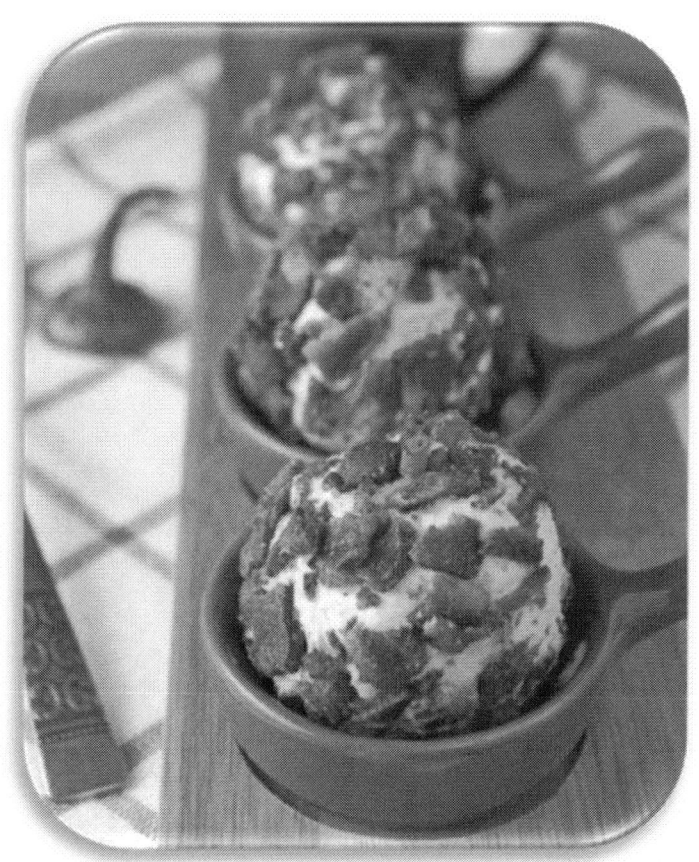

Instructions:

1. Preheat the oven to 325°F. Cook the bacon slices on a baking sheet for 30 minutes. Crumble the bacon. Reserve the bacon grease.
2. In a skillet, heat half of the butter. Add the livers. Cook for 5 minutes. Transfer to a blender and pulse.
3. In another skillet, combine the remaining butter, onion, and garlic. Cook for 10 minutes. Transfer to a blender, add the bacon grease and the remaining ingredients except for the bacon and pulse. Refrigerate for 30 minutes.
4. Make 6 fat bombs from the mixture. Roll them in the crumbled bacon. Serve or store in the fridge for up to 5 days.

Salmon & Dill Fat Bombs

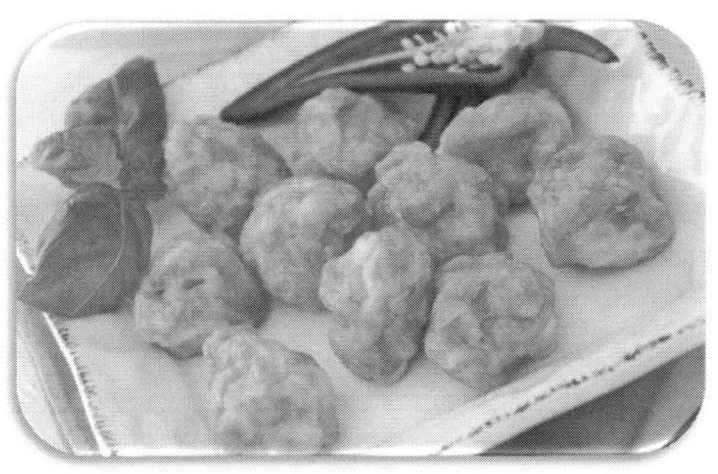

Prep time: 5 min (+ 30 min)

Cooking time: 0 min

Servings: 12

Nutrients per serving:

Total Carbs – 1.4 g

Net Carbs – 0.3 g

Fat –13.4 g

Protein – 3 g

Calories – 174

Ingredients:

- 1 cup cream cheese
- 2/3 cup butter
- ½ package (2 oz) of smoked salmon
- Lemon juice to taste
- Dill to taste
- Salt to taste

Instructions:

1. Place all ingredients in a food processor and blend.
2. Create small balls with the mixture and put in the refrigerator for 30 minutes. Serve cold.

Buttered Bacon Fat Bomb

Prep time: 2 min

Cooking time: 0 min

Servings: 1

Nutrients per serving:

Total Carbs –0.7 g

Net Carbs – 0.5 g

Fat –8.1 g

Protein – 0.8 g

Calories – 77

Ingredients:

- 4 bacon slice
- 4 tbsp Kerrygold butter, unsalted
- 1 tsp garlic powder
- 1/3 cup pecans, toasted, chopped

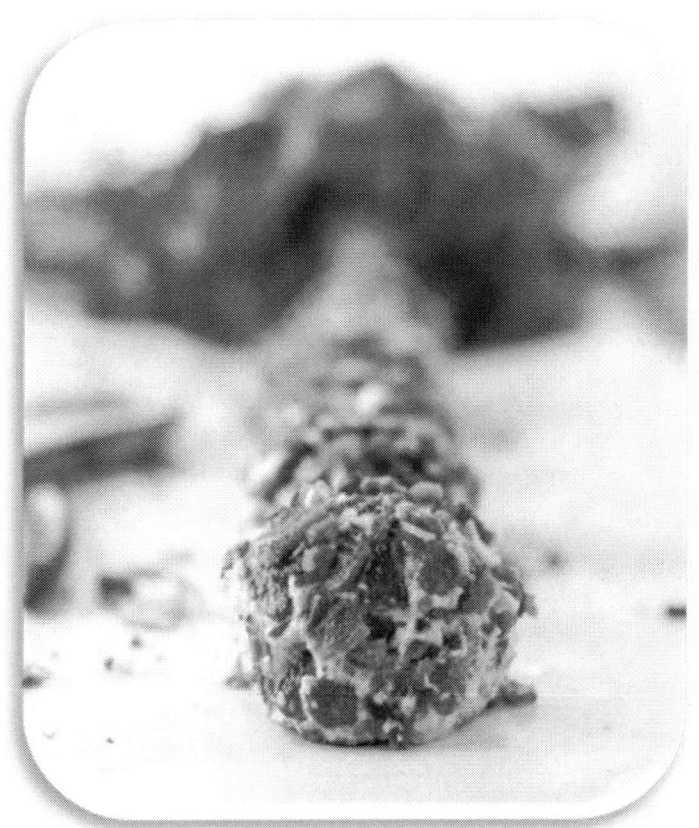

Instructions:

1. Preheat the oven to 325°F. Cook the bacon slice on a baking sheet for 30 minutes. Crumble the bacon.
2. In a bowl, mix remaining ingredients. Refrigerate for 15 mins.
3. Make 4 fat bombs out of the mixture. Roll each fat bomb in the crumbled bacon. Serve or store in the fridge.

Sesame Fat Bombs

Prep time: 15 min (+ 15 min)

Cooking time: 0 min

Servings: 4

Nutrients per serving:

Total Carbs – 0 g

Net Carbs – 0 g

Fat –4.5 g

Protein – 2 g

Calories – 123

Ingredients:

- 4 oz butter
- 2 tbsp sesame oil
- 1 tsp sea salt
- ¼ tsp chili flakes
- 2 tsp sesame seeds, toasted

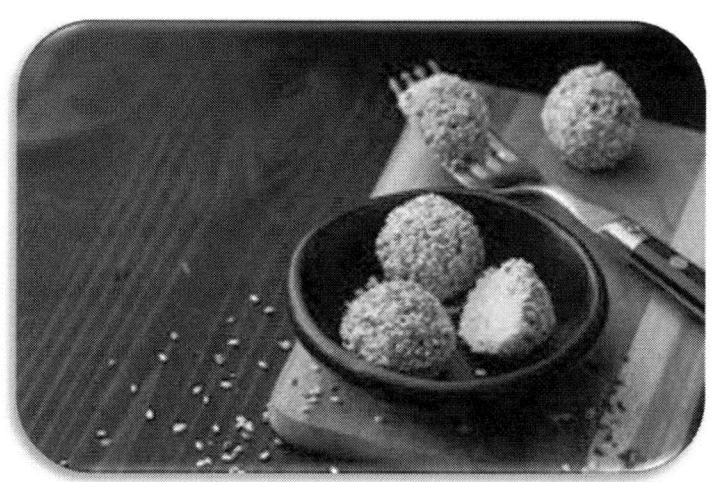

Instructions:

1. In a pan, toast sesame seeds 5 minutes. Set aside.
2. In a bowl, mix remaining ingredients. Refrigerate for 15 mins.
3. Make 4 fat bombs out of the mixture. Roll each fat bomb in the toasted sesame seeds. Serve or store in the fridge.

Keto Cheese Meatballs

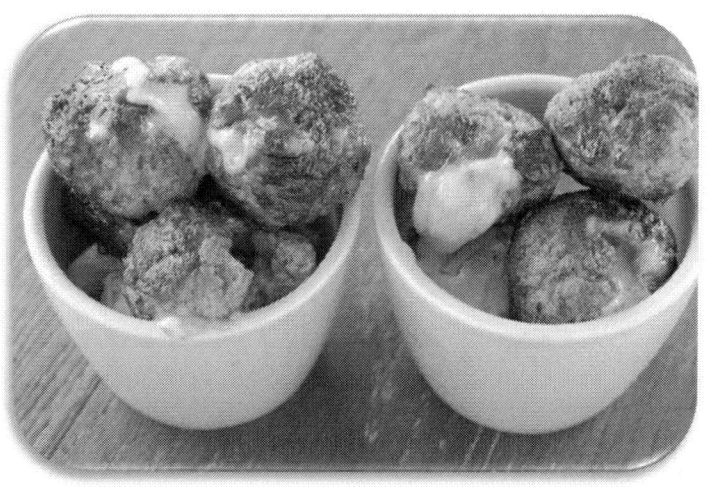

Prep time: 10 min

Cooking time: 10 min

Servings: 9

Nutrients per serving:

Total Carbs – 3.6 g

Net Carbs – 2 g

Fat – 28 g

Protein – 46 g

Calories – 444

Ingredients:

- 17 oz beef, ground
- 4 oz mozzarella cheese
- 3 tbsp Parmesan cheese
- 1 tsp garlic powder
- 3 tbsp olive oil
- Salt, pepper to taste

Instructions:

1. Cut the cheese into cubes.
2. Combine the dry ingredients with the ground beef.
3. Roll the cubes of cheese with the beef, making 9 balls.
4. Fry the meatballs in olive oil for 10 minutes. Let chill and serve.

Keto Scotch Eggs

Prep time: 15 min

Cooking time: 20 min

Servings: 6

Nutrients per serving:

Total Carbs – 0.5 g

Net Carbs – 0.2 g

Fat – 22.5 g

Protein – 28.2 g

Calories – 319

Ingredients:

- 6 eggs, boiled
- 1 lb 2 oz pork, ground
- 2 tsp herbs of choice
- 1 tsp onion flakes
- Salt and pepper to taste

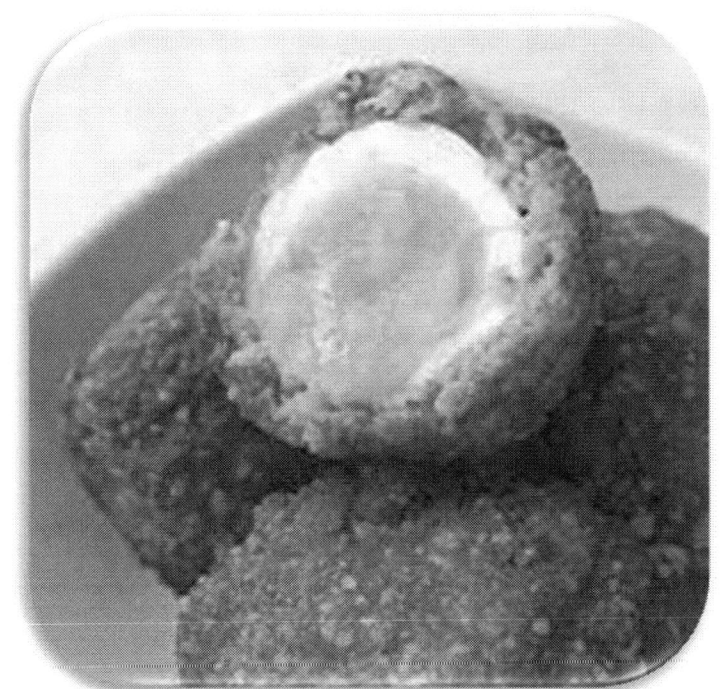

Instructions:

1. Hard-boil the eggs and remove the shells
2. Combine the ground meat, the herbs, spices, and salt and pepper.
3. Coat each egg with enough meat mixture to cover.
4. Sprinkle Scotch eggs with oil in a lined baking tray.
5. Bake at 350°F for 20 minutes. or until golden on all sides. Cool and serve.

Keto Sausage Balls

Prep time: 10 min

Cooking time: 20 min

Servings: 20

Nutrients per serving:

Total Carbs – 1 g

Net Carbs – 0.2 g

Fat – 11 g

Protein – 6 g

Calories – 124

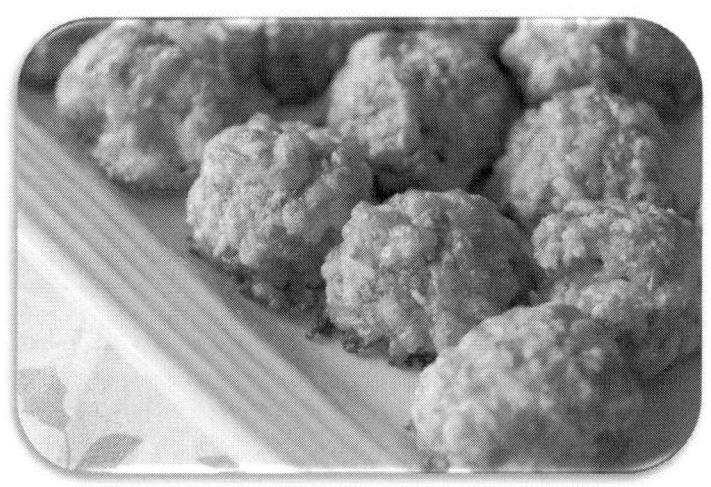

Ingredients:

- 1 lb breakfast sausage,
- 1 egg
- 1 cup almond flour
- 8 oz Cheddar cheese, grated
- ¼ cup Parmesan, grated
- 1 tbsp butter
- 2 tsp baking powder

Instructions:

1. Preheat oven to 350°F
2. Mix all ingredients in a large bowl.
3. Make 20 sausage balls out of the mixture. Put sausage balls on a baking sheet.
4. Bake for 20 minutes. Serve.

Cheesy Jalapeño Fat Bombs

Prep time: 20 min (+ 1 hr)

Cooking time: 30 min

Servings: 6

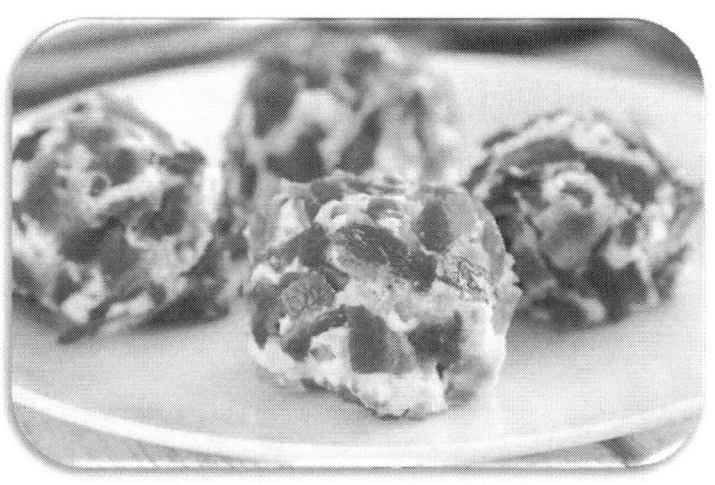

Nutrients per serving:

Total Carbs – 0.9 g

Net Carbs – 0.7 g

Fat – 15 g

Protein – 3.5 g

Calories – 142

Ingredients:

- 3,5 oz full-fat cream cheese
- ¼ cup unsalted butter
- 4 bacon slices
- ¼ cup Cheddar cheese, grated
- 2 jalapeño peppers, seeded, chopped

Instructions:

1. Prchcat the oven to 325°F. Line a baking sheet with parchment paper.
2. Lay the bacon slices on the parchment. Cook for 30 minutes. in the oven. Crumble the bacon into a bowl. Reserve the grease.
3. Blend together the cream cheese and butter. Transfer to a bowl.
4. Add the Cheddar cheese, jalapeños, and bacon grease. Mix well. Refrigerate for 1 hour.
5. Make 6 fat bombs out of the mixture. Roll them in the bacon crumbs. Refrigirate for 1 hour. Serve.

Avocado & Egg Fat Bombs

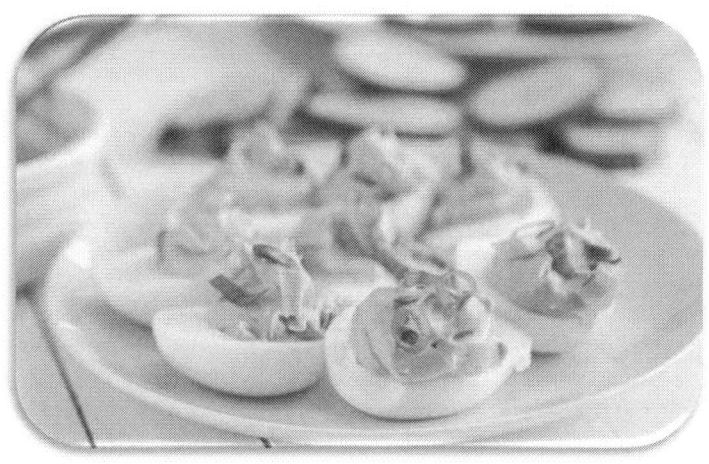

Prep time: 20 min (+ 1 hr)

Cooking time: 0 min

Servings: 2

Nutrients per serving:

Total Carbs – 2.5 g

Net Carbs – 1.1 g

Fat –14.8 g

Protein – 2.2 g

Calories – 147

Ingredients:

- 3 large cooked egg yolks
- ½ avocado, peeled, pitted and chopped
- ¼ cup mayonnaise
- 1 tbsp lemon juice
- 2 tbsp spring onions, chopped
- Salt, pepper to taste

Instructions:

1. Boil the eggs for 10 minutes.
2. Halve the eggs. Scoop the egg yolks into a bowl.
3. Blend chopped avocado and the remaining ingredients in a food processor.
4. Mix the avocado mixture with the egg yolks.
5. Enjoy with cucumber slices and chopped spring onion on top, or fill up the egg white halves and make deviled eggs. Serve.

Savory Salmon Bites

Prep time: 5 min (+ 2 hr)

Cooking time: 0 min

Servings: 12

Nutrients per serving:

Total Carbs – 1 g

Net Carbs – 1 g

Fat – 13 g

Protein – 3 g

Calories – 117

Ingredients:

- 2 oz smoked salmon trimmings.
- 1 cup mascarpone cheese
- 2/3 cup grass-fed butter, softened
- 1 tbsp apple cider vinegar
- 1 tbsp chopped parsley
- Salt to taste

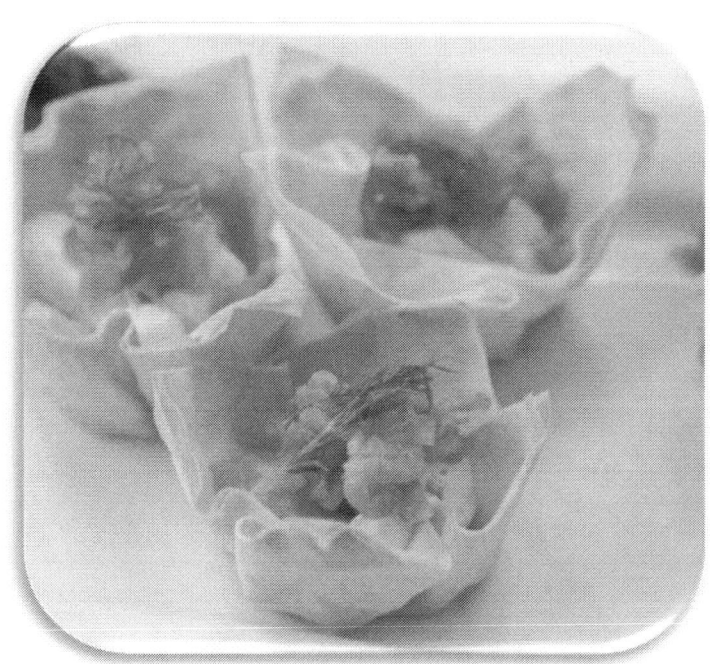

Instructions:

1. Smash the cheese with a fork to soften and add the remaining ingredients.
2. Form into small balls, and place on a tray lined with parchment paper.
3. Put in the fridge for 2 hours. Serve.

Savory Salmon Fat Bombs

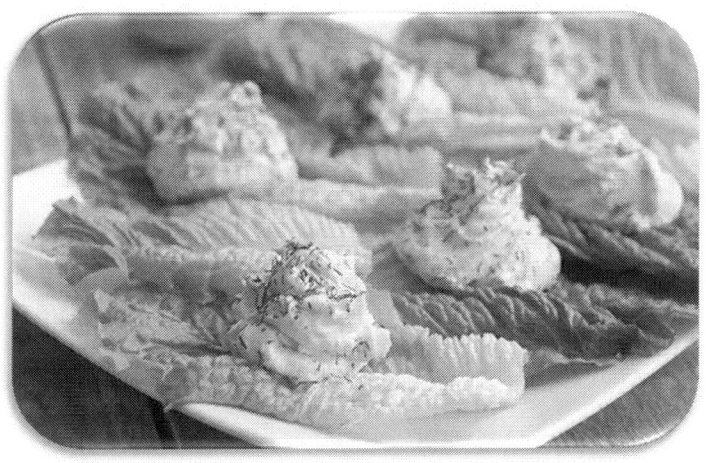

Prep time: 10 min (+ 2 hr)

Cooking time: 0 min

Servings: 6

Nutrients per serving:

Total Carbs – 0.8 g

Net Carbs – 0.7 g

Fat – 15.7 g

Protein – 3.2 g

Calories – 147

Ingredients:

- ½ cup full-fat cream cheese
- 1/3 cup butter, grass-fed
- ½ package (2 oz) smoked salmon
- 1 tbsp fresh lemon juice
- 1-2 tbsp dill, chopped
- 5 lettuce leaves

Instructions:

1. Pulse all ingredients together in a food processor.
2. Line a tray with parchment paper and make fat bombs using about 2½ tbsp of the mixture for each. Refrigerate for 2 hours, garnish with more dill and place on top of lettuce leaves.
3. Serve or store in an airtight container in the fridge for up to a week.

Cheesy Pesto Fat Bombs

Prep time: 5 min (+ 2 hr)

Cooking time: 0 min

Servings: 6

Nutrients per serving:

Total Carbs – 1.6 g

Net Carbs – 1.3 g

Fat –12.9 g

Protein – 4.3 g

Calories – 123

Ingredients:

- 1 cup full-fat cream cheese
- 2 tbsp basil pesto
- ½ cup Parmesan cheese, grated
- 10 green olives, sliced
- 6 cucumber slices

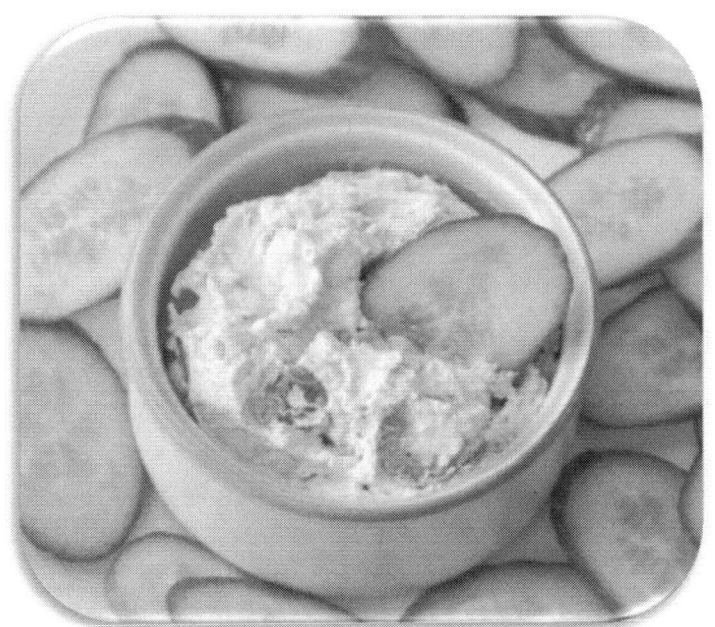

Instructions:

1. Using a spatula, mix all the ingredients in a bowl until well combined.
2. Serve as a dip with sliced cucumber or other fresh vegetables.
3. You can also refrigerate for 30 minutes, then create balls and roll in Parmesan cheese.
4. Serve as a dip with cucumber slices.

Herbed Cheese Fat Bombs

Prep time: 10 min (+ 30 min)

Cooking time: 0 min

Servings: 5

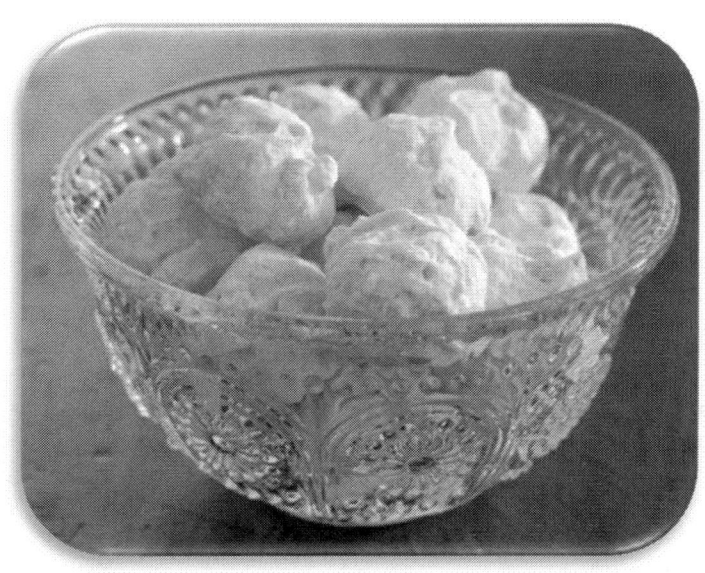

Nutrients per serving:

Total Carbs – 2 g

Net Carbs – 1.7 g

Fat – 17.1 g

Protein – 3.7 g

Calories – 164

Ingredients:

- 3.5 oz full-fat cream cheese
- ¼ cup unsalted butter
- 4 pieces sun-dried tomatoes, drained, chopped
- 4 pitted green olives, chopped
- 2 tsp dried herbs
- 2 garlic cloves, crushed
- 5 tbsp Parmesan cheese, grated
- Salt, pepper to taste

Instructions:

1. Blend together the cream cheese and butter. Transfer to a bowl.
2. Add the next four ingredients. Season with salt and pepper, and mix. Refrigerate for 30 minutes.
3. Make 5 balls out of the mixture. Roll each ball in the Parmesan cheese. Serve.

Pork Belly Fat Bombs

Prep time: 10 min (+ 30 min)

Cooking time: 0 min

Servings: 6

Nutrients per serving:

Total Carbs – 0.5 g

Net Carbs – 0.3 g

Fat – 26.4 g

Protein – 3.5 g

Calories – 263

Ingredients:

- 3 bacon slices, cut in half widthwise
- 5.3 oz pork belly, cooked
- ¼ cup mayonnaise
- 1 tbsp Dijon mustard
- 1 tbsp fresh horseradish, grated
- Salt, pepper to taste
- 6 lettuce leaves, for serving

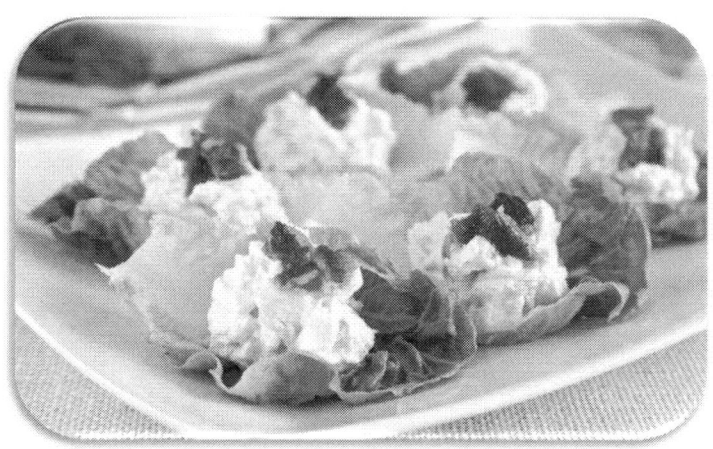

Instructions:

1. Preheat the oven to 325°F.
2. Cook the bacon slices on a baking sheet for 30 minutes. in the oven. Let cool.
3. Crumble the bacon into a dish and set aside.
4. Shred the pork belly into a bowl. Mix in the mayonnaise, mustard, and horseradish. Season with salt and pepper.
5. Divide the mixture into 6 mounds. Top with the crumbled bacon and serve on top of lettuce leaves.

Veggie & Cheese Fat Bombs

Prep time: 15 min (+ 30 min)

Cooking time: 6 min

Servings: 6

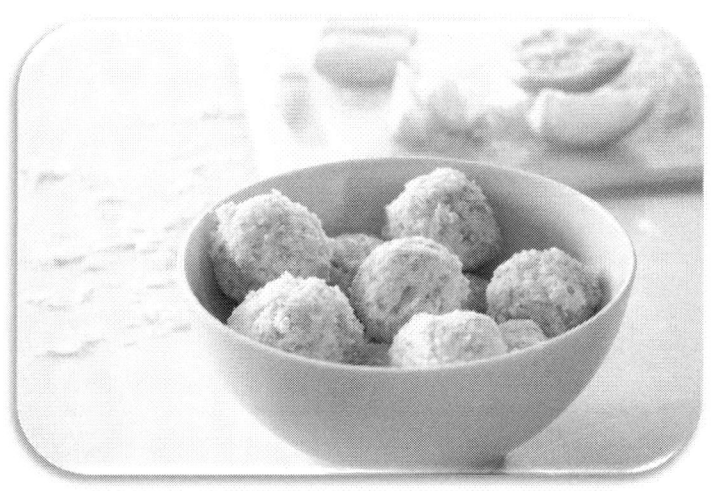

Nutrients per serving:

Total Carbs – 3.6 g

Net Carbs – 3 g

Fat –16.7 g

Protein – 3.4 g

Calories – 166

Ingredients:

- 3.5 oz full-fat cream cheese,
- ¼ cup unsalted butter
- 1 tbsp ghee
- ½ onion, peeled, chopped
- 1 garlic clove, peeled and finely chopped
- ½ cup dried porcini mushrooms
- 2 cups spinach
- Salt, pepper to taste
- ¼ cup hard goat cheese, grated

Instructions:

1. Mix the cream cheese and butter in a food processor.
2. In a pan, cook the onion and garlic with ghee over medium heat for 3 minutes. Add the dried chopped mushrooms and spinach; cook for another 3 min. Set aside to cool.
3. Mix the cream cheese and butter with the cooled mushroom and spinach mixture. Season with salt and pepper. Refrigerate for 30 minutes.
4. Make 5 balls out of the mixture. Roll each ball in the goat cheese. Serve.

Ham & Cheese Fat Bombs

Prep time: 15 min (+ 30 min)

Cooking time: 0 min

Servings: 6

Nutrients per serving:

Total Carbs – 0.9 g

Net Carbs – 0.7 g

Fat – 16.7 g

Protein – 6.4 g

Calories – 167

Ingredients:

- 3.5 oz full-fat cream cheese
- ¼ cup unsalted butter
- ¼ cup Cheddar cheese, grated
- 2 tbsp fresh basil, chopped
- 6 slices Parma ham
- 6 large green olives, pitted
- Pepper to taste

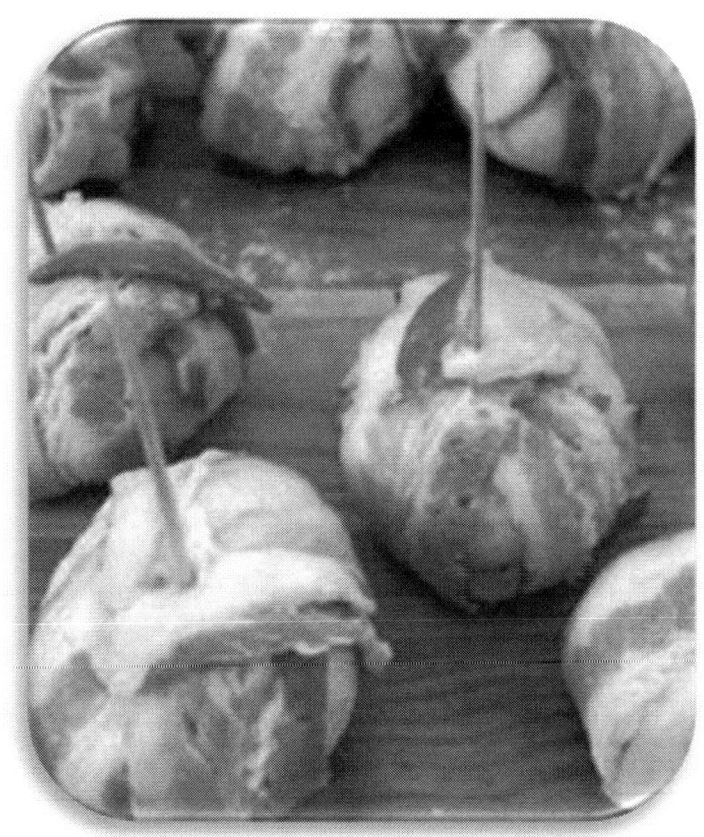

Instructions:

1. In a food processor, blend the cream cheese and butter.
2. Add the Cheddar cheese and basil, mix well. Season with pepper. Refrigerate for 30 minutes.
3. Make 6 balls out of the mixture. Roll each ball with 1 slice of Parma ham, top with 1 olive, piercing it with a toothpick. Serve.

Tomato & Olive Fat Bombs

Prep time: 15 min (+ 30 min)

Cooking time: 0 min

Servings: 6

Nutrients per serving:

Total Carbs – 3 g

Fiber – 1.1 g

Net Carbs – 1.9 g

Fat –18.1 g

Protein – 4.2 g

Calories – 178

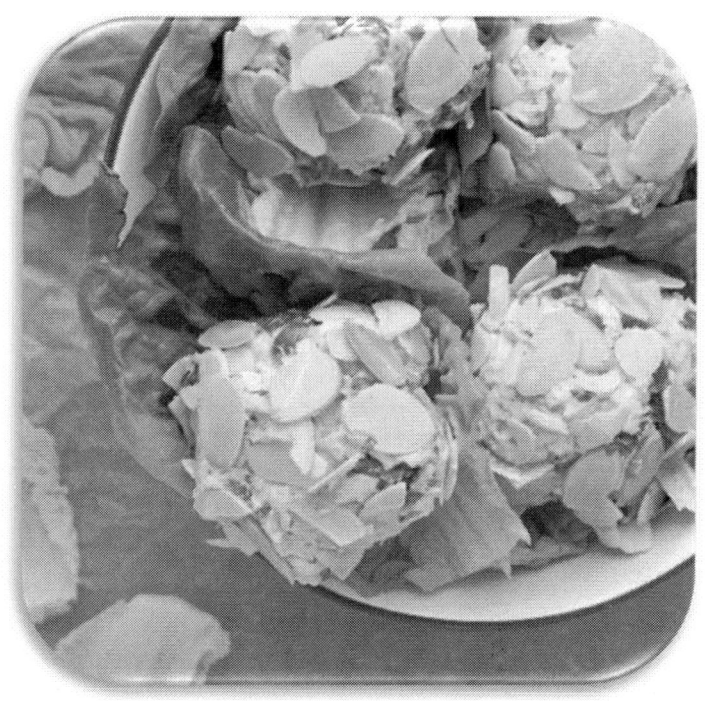

Ingredients:

- 3.5 oz full-fat cream cheese
- ¼ cup unsalted butter
- ¼ cup Manchego cheese, grated
- ¼ cup sun-dried tomatoes, drained, chopped
- ¼ cup green olives, pitted, sliced
- 2 tbsp capers, drained
- 1 garlic clove, crushed
- 1/3 cup flaked almonds, raw or toasted
- Pepper to taste

Instructions:

1. In a food processor, blend the cream cheese and butter until smooth.
2. Add the next five ingredients. Season with pepper. Mix well. Refrigerate for 30 minutes.
3. Make 6 balls out of the mixture. Roll each ball in the almond flakes. Serve.

Stilton & Chive Fat Bombs

Prep time: 15 min (+ 30 min)

Cooking time: 0 min

Servings: 6

Nutrients per serving:

Total Carbs – 1.1 g

Fiber – 0.2 g

Net Carbs – 0.8 g

Fat –16.2 g

Protein – 5 g

Calories – 157

Ingredients:

- 3.5 oz full-fat cream cheese
- ¼ cup unsalted butter
- ½ cup Stilton, crumbled
- 2 spring onions, chopped
- 1 tbsp parsley, chopped
- 1/3 cup fresh chives, chopped

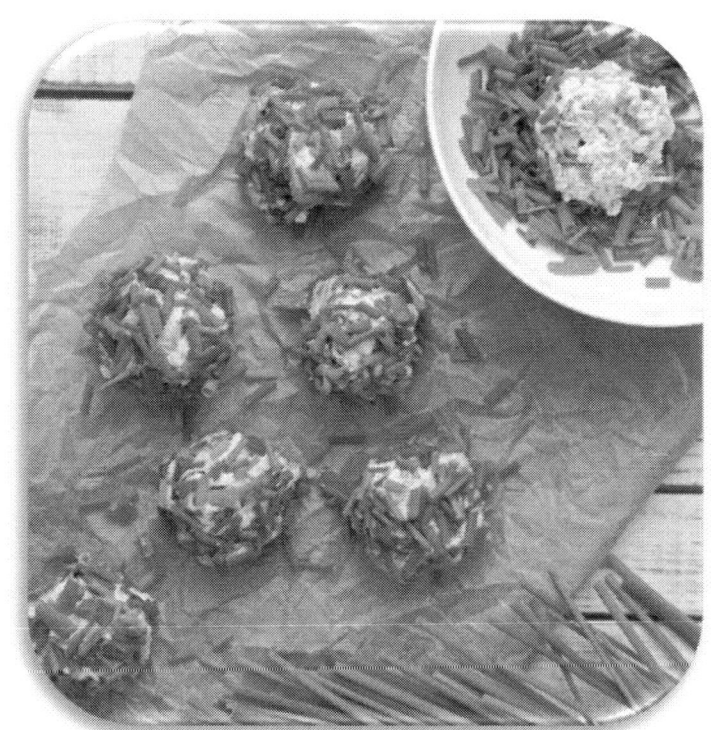

Instructions:

1. In a food processor, mix the cream cheese and butter.
2. Add the crumbled blue cheese, spring onions, and parsley. Mix well. Refrigerate for 30 minutes.
3. Make 6 balls out of the mixture. Roll each ball in the chives. Serve.

Easy Savory Fat Bombs

Prep time: 20 min (+ 1 hr)

Cooking time: 30 min

Servings: 6

Nutrients per serving:

Total Carbs – 0.9 g

Net Carbs – 0.8 g

Fat –14.6 g

Protein – 2.7 g

Calories – 136

Ingredients:

- 3.5 oz full-fat cream cheese
- ¼ cup unsalted butter
- 2 bacon slices
- 1 garlic clove, crushed
- 1 spring onion, sliced
- Salt, pepper to taste
- 6 lettuce leaves

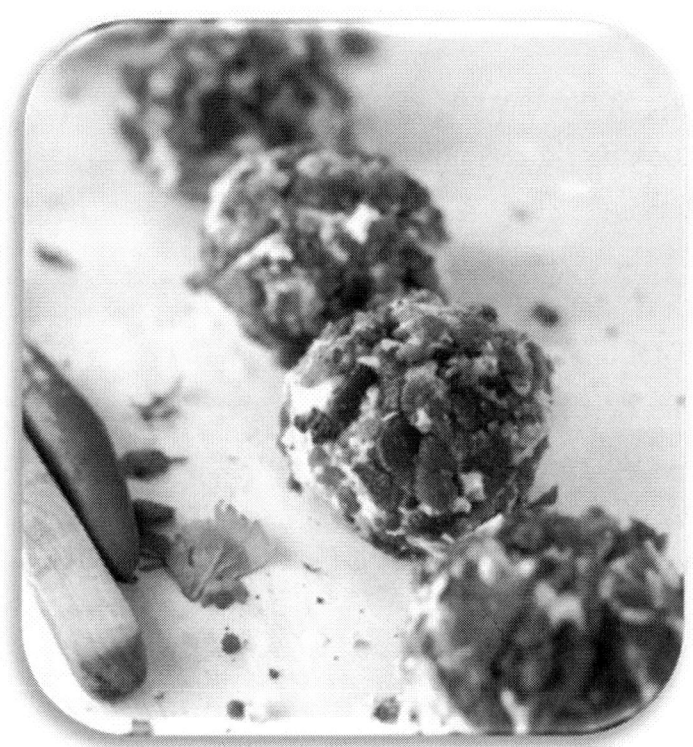

Instructions:

1. In a food processor, mix the cream cheese and butter. Transfer to a bowl.
2. Preheat the oven to 325°F.
3. Cook the bacon slices on a baking sheet for 30 minutes. Reserve the grease and crumble the bacon in a bowl.
4. Add the garlic, sliced onion, bacon (reserve some for later), and bacon grease from the sheet to the bowl with the butter mixture. Season with salt and pepper. Mix well. Refrigerate for 1 hour.
5. Make 6 fat bombs out of the mixture. Roll them in reserved crumbled bacon. Serve.

Brie Cheese Fat Bombs

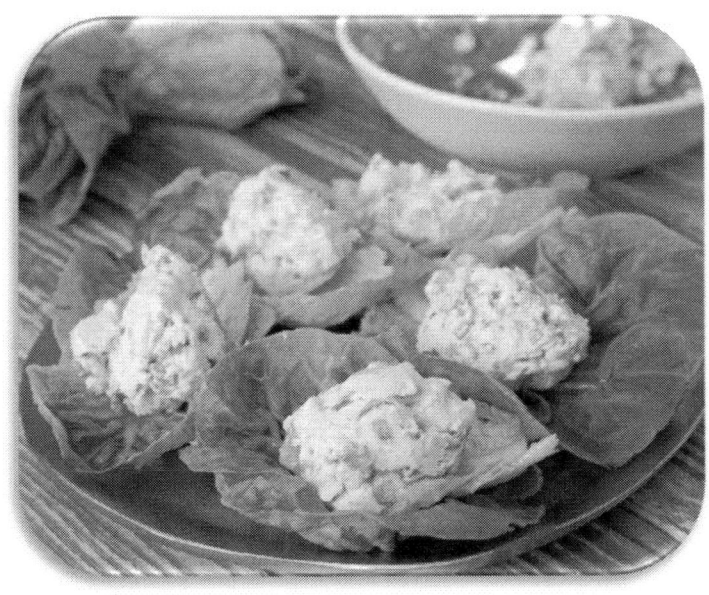

Prep time: 15 min (+ 30 min)

Cooking time: 3 min

Servings: 6

Nutrients per serving:

Total Carbs – 1.7 g

Fiber – 0.3 g

Net Carbs –1.4 g

Fat –16.2 g

Protein – 3.3 g

Calories – 158

Ingredients:

- 2 oz full-fat cream cheese
- ¼ cup unsalted butter
- ½ cup Brie cheese, chopped
- 1 tbsp ghee
- 1 white onion, diced
- 1 garlic clove, minced
- ½ tsp paprika
- Salt, pepper to taste
- 6 lettuce leaves

Instructions:

1. In a food processor, mix the cream cheese and butter. Transfer to a bowl. Mix in the Brie.
2. In a pan, add onion and garlic and cook 3 minutes over medium heat with ghee. Let cool. Once cooled, combine with the cheese and butter mixture.
3. Season with the spices and mix. Refrigerate 30 minutes.
4. Make 6 fat bombs out of the mixture. Serve on lettuce leaves.

Bacon, Artichoke & Onion Fat Bombs

Prep time: 15 min (+ 30 min)

Cooking time: 8 min

Servings: 4

Nutrients per serving:

Total Carbs – 10 g

Net Carbs – 4 g

Fat – 39.6 g

Protein – 6.6 g

Calories – 408

Ingredients:

- 2 bacon slices
- 2 tbsp ghee
- ½ large onion, peeled, diced
- 1 garlic clove, minced
- 1/3 cup canned artichoke hearts, sliced
- ¼ cup sour cream
- ¼cup mayonnaise
- 1 tbsp lemon juice
- ¼ cup Swiss cheese, grated
- Salt, pepper to taste
- 4 avocado halves, pitted

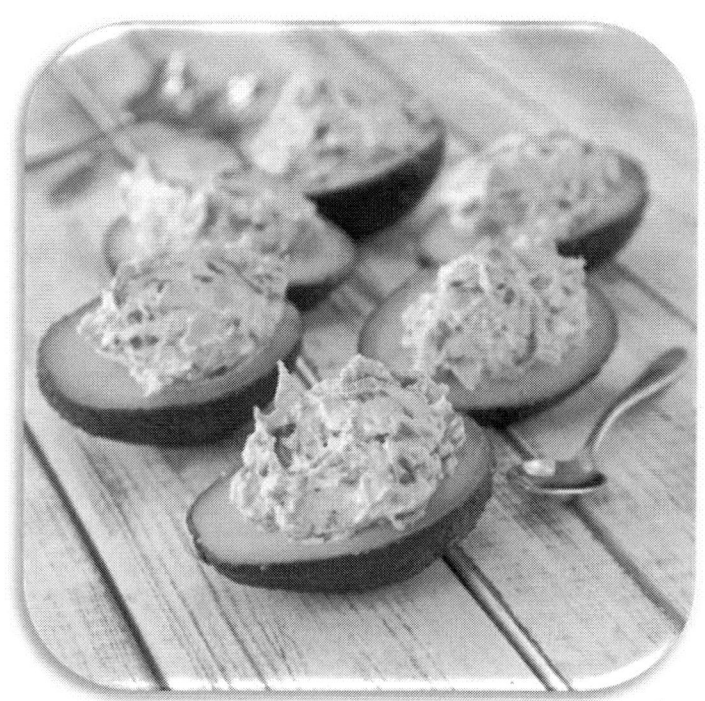

Instructions:

1. In a hot skillet, fry the bacon for 5 minutes. Let cool, then crumble.
2. Cook the onion and garlic using ghee for 3 minutes.
3. Combine the onion and garlic with the bacon and the remaining ingredients. Mix well. Season with salt and pepper. Refrigerate 30 minutes. Fill the avocado halves with the mixture and serve.

Chorizo & Avocado Fat Bombs

Prep time: 15 min (+ 30 min)

Cooking time: 8 min

Servings: 4

Nutrients per serving:

Total Carbs – 9.5 g

Net Carbs – 2.7 g

Fat – 38.9 g

Protein – 11.4 g

Calories – 419

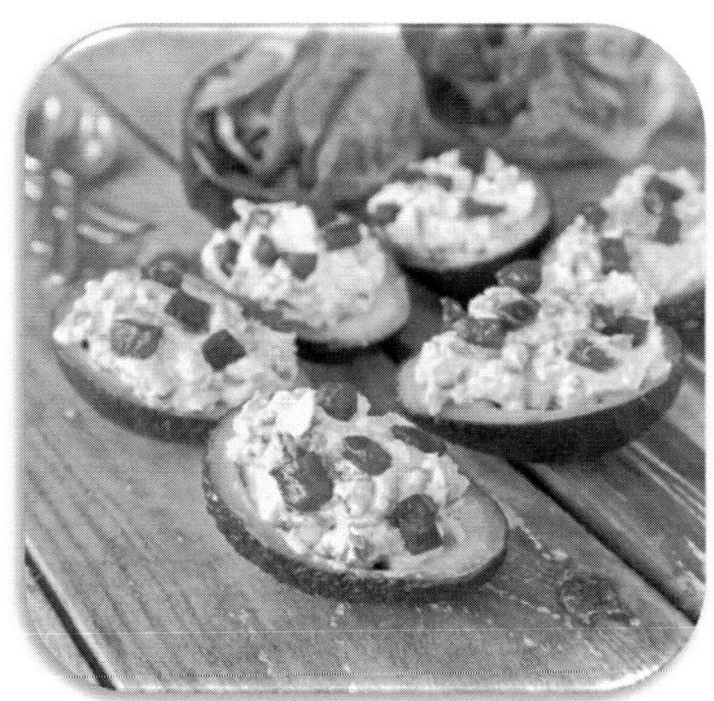

Ingredients:

- 3. 5 oz Spanish chorizo sausage, diced
- 2 large hard-boiled eggs, diced
- ¼ cup unsalted butter
- 2 tbsp mayonnaise
- 1 tbsp lemon juice
- 2 tbsp chives, chopped
- Salt, cayenne pepper to taste
- 4 avocado halves, pitted

Instructions:

1. In a hot pan, fry the chorizo for 5 minutes. Set aside.
2. In a mixing bowl, combine all ingredients. Season with salt and cayenne pepper. Mash together with a fork. Refrigerate for 30 minutes, and then fill each avocado half with ¼ of the mixture.
3. Serve one-quarter of the mixture on top of each avocado half.

Bacon Ranch Fat Bombs

Prep time: 15 min (+ 2 hr)

Cooking time: 15 min

Servings: 4

Nutrients per serving:

Total Carbs – 9.5 g

Fiber – 6.8 g

Net Carbs – 2.7 g

Fat – 38.9 g

Protein – 11.4 g

Calories – 419

Ingredients:

- 8 oz full-fat cream cheese, softened
- 1 tbsp ranch dressing dry mix
- 2 slices bacon

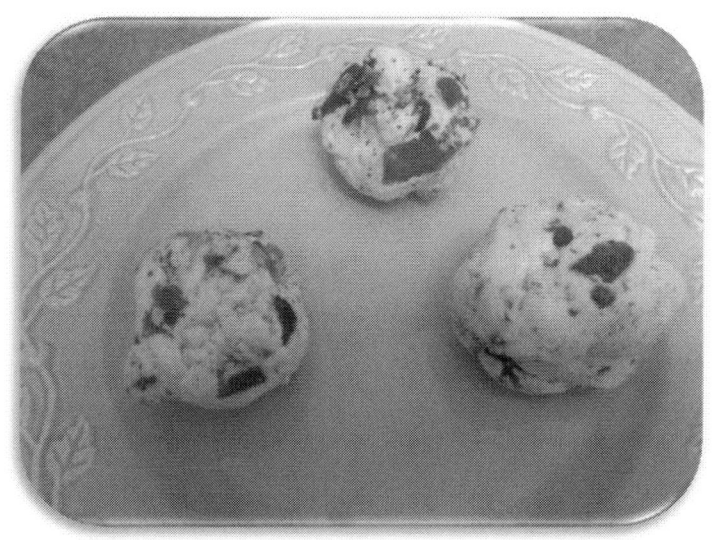

Instructions:

1. Preheat the oven to 375°F.
2. Cook the bacon strips on a baking tray for 15 minutes. Let cool, then crumble.
3. In a bowl, add cream cheese and sprinkle with ranch dressing dry mix. Stir in the bacon. Mix thoroughly.
4. Form a ball out of 1 tbsp of the mixture. Repeat to form 3 more bombs. Refrigerate for 2 hours. Serve.

Crispy Bacon Fat Bombs

Prep time: 10 min (+30 min)

Cooking time: 3 min

Servings: 4

Nutrients per serving:

Total Carbs – 1.4 g

Net Carbs – 0.5 g

Fat – 12.9 g

Protein – 5.7 g

Calories – 141

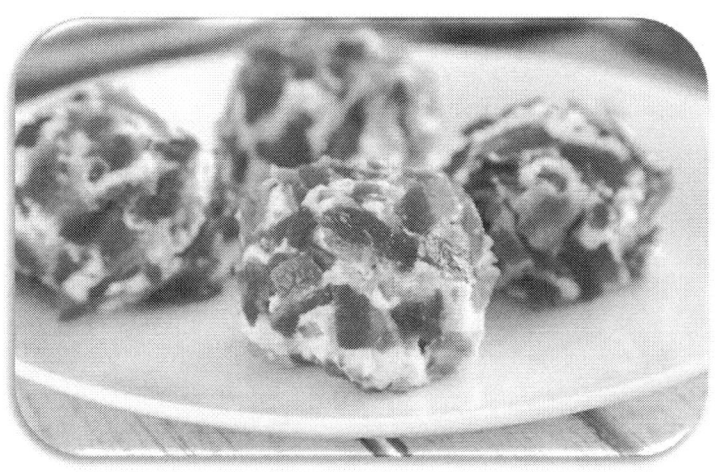

Ingredients:

- 4 thick bacon slices
- 4 oz cream cheese
- 1 green chile, seeded, chopped
- 1 tsp onion powder
- Salt and pepper to taste

Instructions:

1. Cook the bacon in a skillet for 3 minutes. Let cool, then crumble. Reserve the bacon fat.
2. In a bowl, combine the remaining ingredients. Add the bacon fat and mix.
3. Shape the mixture into 4 fat bombs. Refrigirate for 30 min.
4. Roll the fat bombs in the crumbled bacon. Serve.

SWEET FAT BOMBS

Orange & Walnut Chocolate Fat Bombs

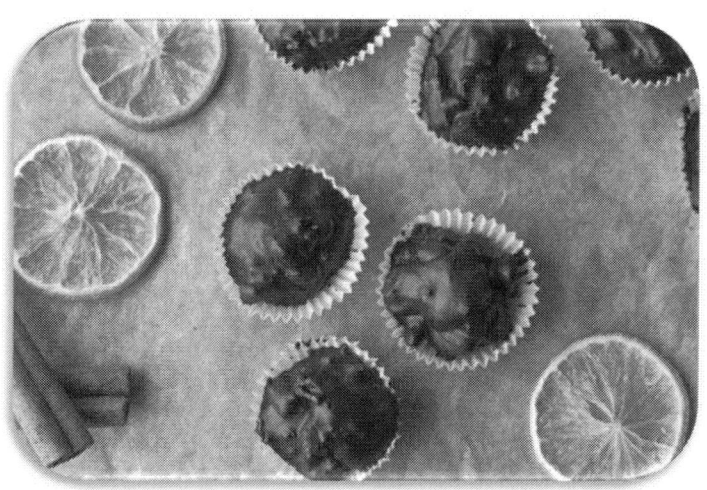

Prep time: 20 min (+ 2 hr)

Cooking time: 0 min

Servings: 8

Nutrients per serving:

Total Carbs – 2.4 g

Net Carbs – 1.5 g

Fat – 8.4 g

Protein – 1.5 g

Calories – 87

Ingredients:

- 4.5 oz dark chocolate, 85% cocoa
- ¼ cup extra-virgin coconut oil
- 11/3 cups walnuts, chopped
- 1 tbsp orange peel
- 1 tsp cinnamon
- 15 drops of stevia

Instructions:

1. Melt the chocolate in a double boiler. Mix in the other ingredients.
2. Transfer the mixture into 8 small paper muffin or candy cups.
3. Refrigerate for 2 hours. Serve.

Keto Chocolate Coconut Candies

Prep time: 20 min (+ 55 min)

Cooking time: 0 min

Servings: 9

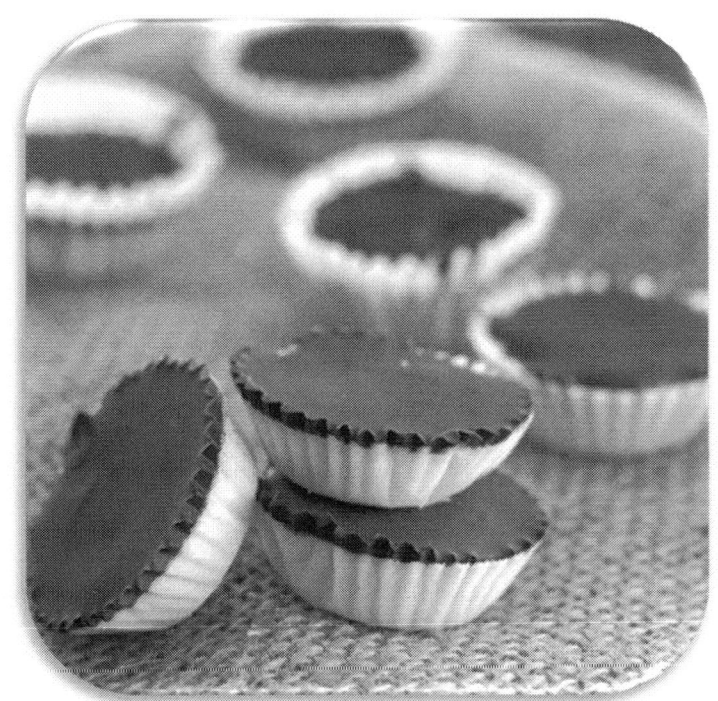

Nutrients per serving:

Total Carbs – 2.4 g

Net Carbs – 1 g

Fat –7.7 g

Protein – 0.92 g

Calories – 76

Ingredients:

- 1 cup extra-virgin coconut oil
- 1 cup cocoa powder
- 1 tsp vanilla bean powder
- ¼ cup powdered erythritol.
- 15 drops stevia extract
- Salt to taste
- ¼ cup coconut butter, chilled

Instructions:

1. Melt coconut oil in a microwave. Combine with the next four ingredients.
2. Spoon about half of the chocolate mixture into silicone molds. Refrigerate for 15 minutes.
3. Then add ½ tsp coconut butter into the molds.
4. Top with the remaining chocolate mixture and refrigerate for 40 minutes.
5. Serve, or store in the refrigerator in a container.

Keto Coconut Fat Bombs

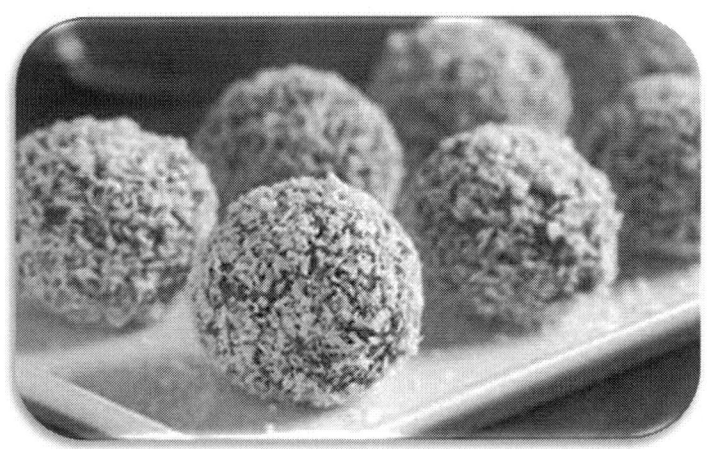

Prep time: 20 min (+ 30 min)

Cooking time: 5 min

Servings: 12

Nutrients per serving:

Total Carbs – 2.6 g

Net Carbs – 0.74 g

Fat – 9.6 g

Protein – 1.9 g

Calories – 104

Ingredients:

- 1½ cups shredded coconut, unsweetened
- ¼ cup extra-virgin coconut oil
- ¼ cup butter, grass-fed
- ¼ tsp cinnamon
- Salt to taste

Instructions:

1. Preheat the oven to 375°F.
2. Toast the coconut on a baking sheet for 5 minutes, and then pulse it in a blender.
3. Add the remaining ingredients and stir thoroughly.
4. Fill 12 mini-muffin forms with 1½ tbsp of the mixture. Refrigerate for 30 minutes. Serve.

Easy Lemon Fat Bombs

Prep time: 15 min (+ 1 hr)

Cooking time: 0 min

Servings: 16

Nutrients per serving:

Total Carbs – 2.9 g

Net Carbs – 0.8 g

Fat – 11.9 g

Protein – 0.76 g

Calories – 112

Ingredients:

- 7 oz coconut butter, softened
- ¼ cup extra-virgin coconut oil, softened
- 1-2 tbsp organic lemon zest, minced
- 20 drops stevia extract

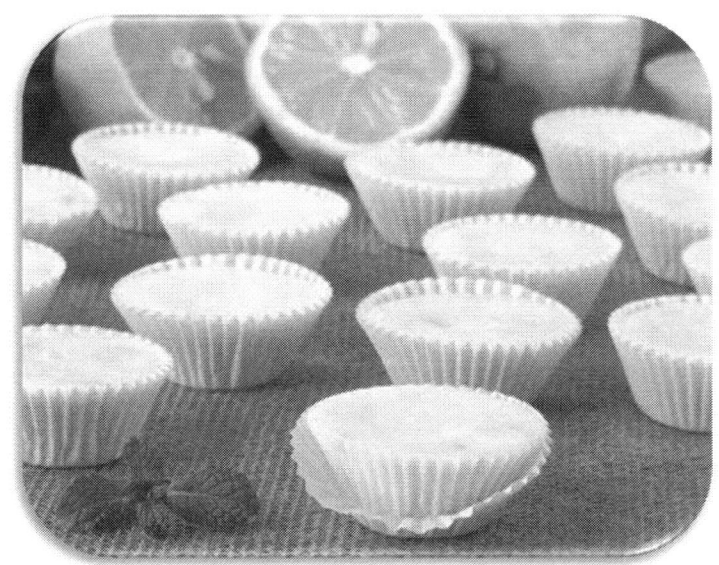

Instructions:

1. In a large bowl, mix all ingredients.
2. Pour 1 tbsp of the coconut mixture into each small muffin paper cup or silicone candy mold and place on a tray. Refrigerate for 1 hour. Serve.

Easy Vanilla Fat Bombs

Prep time: 20 min (+ 30 min)

Cooking time: 0 min

Servings: 14

Nutrients per serving:

Total Carbs – 1.6 g

Fiber – 0.96 g

Net Carbs – 0.6 g

Fat – 14.4 g

Protein – 0.79 g

Calories – 132

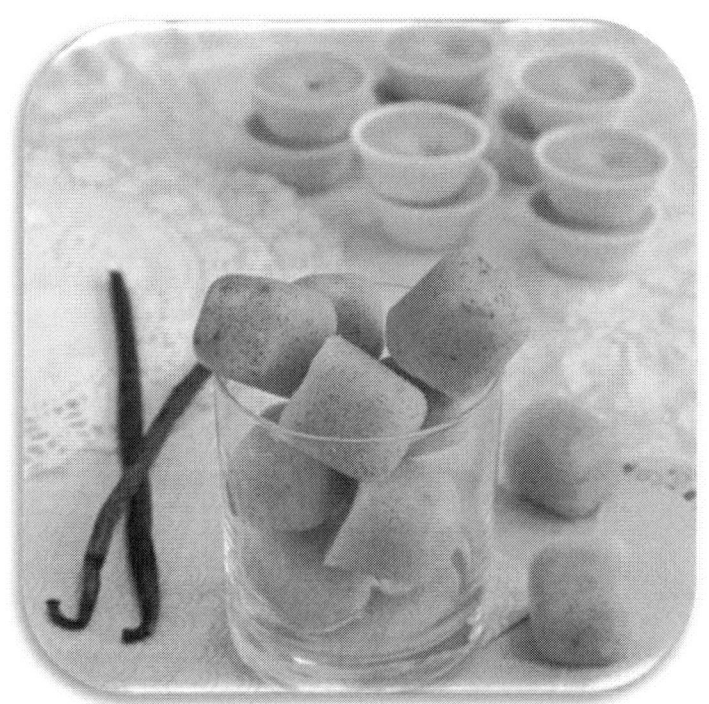

Ingredients:

- 1 cup macadamia nuts, unsalted
- ¼ cup extra-virgin coconut oil
- ¼ cup butter
- 2 tsp sugar-free vanilla extract
- 20 drops stevia extract
- 2 tbsp powdered erythritol

Instructions:

1. Pulse the macadamia nuts in a blender. Combine them with softened butter and coconut oil.
2. Add remaining ingredients. Mix thoroughly.
3. Fill each mini-muffin form with 1½ tbsp of the mixture. Refrigerate for 30 minutes. Serve.

Spiced Cocoa Fat Bombs

Prep time: 10 min (+ 2 hr)

Cooking time: 0 min

Servings: 10

Nutrients per serving:

Total Carbs – 1.8 g

Net Carbs – 1.1 g

Fat – 5 g

Protein – 0.7 g

Calories – 48.8

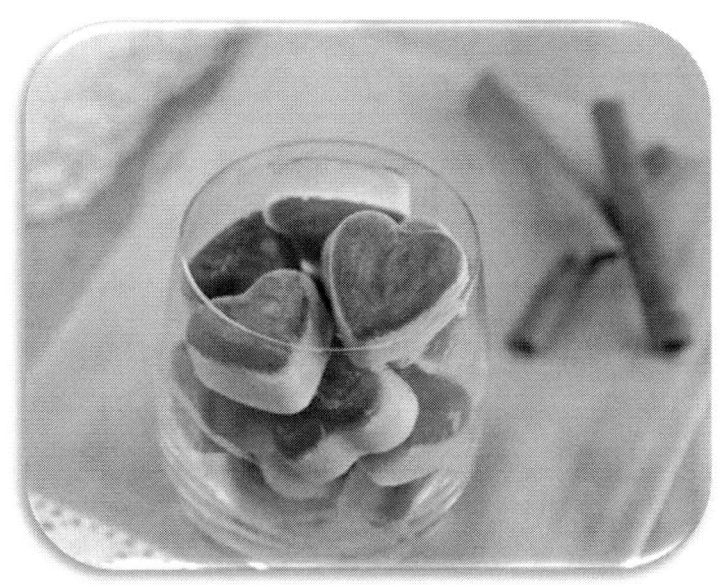

Ingredients:

- 1 cup coconut milk
- 2 tbsp cocoa powder, unsweetened
- 1 tsp vanilla extract, unsweetened
- 1 tsp cinnamon
- ¼ tsp cayenne pepper
- 2 tbsp erythritol
- 20 drops stevia extract

Instructions:

1. Warm the coconut milk.
2. Combine remaining ingredients with coconut milk and mix.
3. Pour the liquid into a heart-shaped form (about 1 tbsp per one). Freeze for 2 hours. Serve.

No Bake Chocolate Peanut Butter Fat Bombs

Prep time: 10 min (+ 20 min)

Cooking time: 0 min

Servings: 8

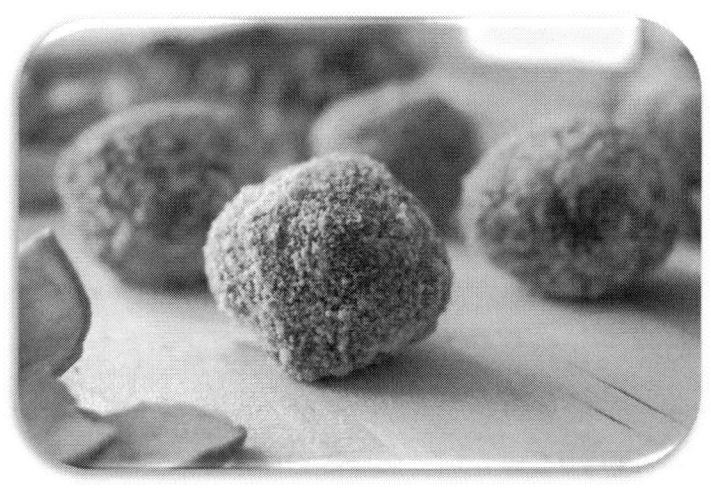

Nutrients per serving:

Total Carbs – 3.1 g

Net Carbs – 0.8 g

Fat – 20 g

Protein – 4.4 g

Calories – 208

Ingredients:

- ½ cup coconut oil
- ¼ cup cocoa powder
- 4 tbsp PB Fit Powder
- 6 tbsp hemp seeds, hulled
- 2 tbsp heavy cream
- 1 tsp vanilla extract
- 28 drops liquid stevia
- ¼ cup coconut, unsweetened, shredded

Instructions:

1. Combine all ingredients except the shredded coconut. Mix to a creamy consistency.
2. Form balls out of the mixture.
3. Roll balls in the coconut. Put them on a baking tray lined with parchment paper. Freeze for about 20 minutes. Serve.

Neapolitan Fat Bombs

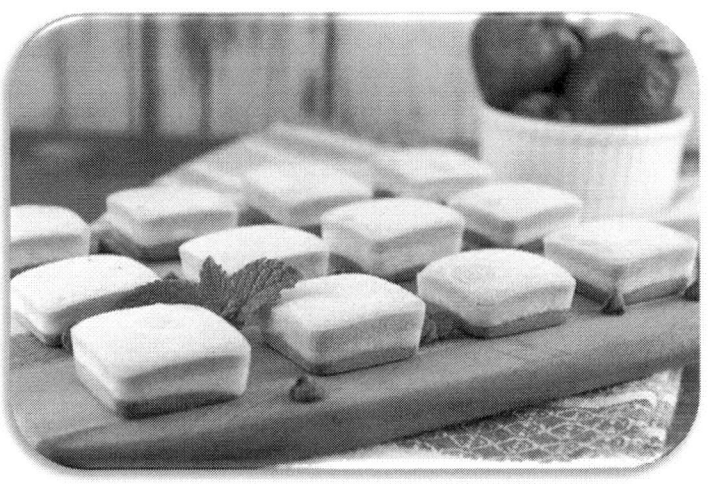

Prep time: 20 min (+ 2 hr 30 min)

Cooking time: 0 min

Servings: 24

Nutrients per serving:

Total Carbs – 0.85 g

Net Carbs – 0.66 g

Fat – 11 g

Protein – 0.51 g

Calories – 102.7

Ingredients:

- ½ cup butter
- ½ cup coconut oil
- ½ cup sour cream
- ½ cup cream cheese
- 2 tbsp erythritol
- 25 drops liquid stevia
- 2 tbsp cocoa powder
- 1 tsp vanilla extract
- 2 strawberries, puréed

Instructions:

1. Blend the first six ingredients.
2. Divide the mixture into 3 different bowls. Stir cocoa powder into the first bowl, strawberries into the second, and vanilla into the third.
3. Pour chocolate mixture into fat bomb mold. Put in freezer for 30 minutes, then repeat with the vanilla mixture Freeze vanilla mixture for 30 minutes, then repeat the process with strawberry mixture.
4. Freeze all again for at least 1 hour. Serve.

Maple Pecan Fat Bomb Bars

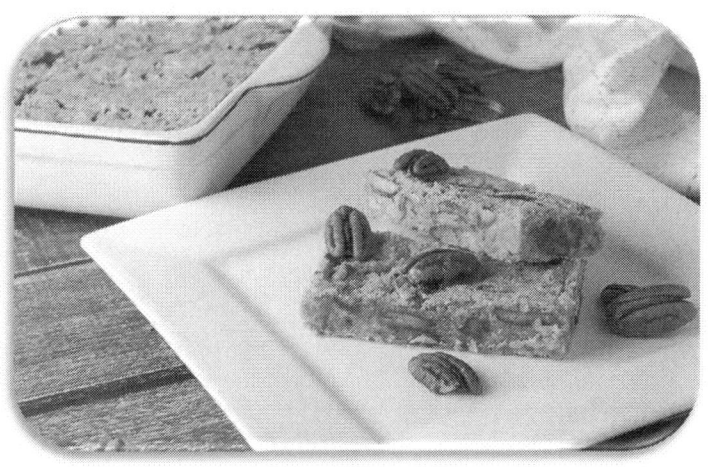

Prep time: 25 min (+ 1 hr)

Cooking time: 30 min

Servings: 12

Nutrients per serving:

Total Carbs – 5.65 g

Net Carbs – 2.51 g

Fat – 29.7 g

Protein – 4.74 g

Calories – 299

Ingredients:

- 2 cups pecan halves
- 1 cup almond flour
- ½ cup golden flaxseed meal
- ½ cup coconut, unsweetened, shredded
- ½ cup coconut oil
- ¼ cup maple syrup
- 25 drops liquid stevia

Instructions:

1. Preheat the oven to 350°F.
2. Toast pecans in the oven for 6-8 minutes. Then cool and crush them in a plastic bag.
3. Mix dry ingredients and pecans together.
4. Mix in remaining ingredients. Make a crumbly dough, spread in a casserole dish and bake for 20-25 minutes at 350°F.
5. Let cool, then refrigerate for 1 hour. Cut into slices and serve

Fall Season Fat Bombs

Prep time: 2 min (+ 2 hr)

Cooking time: 2 min

Servings: 2

Nutrients per serving:

Total Carbs – 4.46 g

Net Carbs – 3.26 g

Fat – 17.8 g

Protein – 3.96 g

Calories – 186

Ingredients:

- 2 tbsp peanut butter
- 1 tbsp heavy cream
- 1 tbsp coconut oil
- 1 tsp cocoa powder
- ¼ tsp allspice
- 4-5 drops liquid sucralose

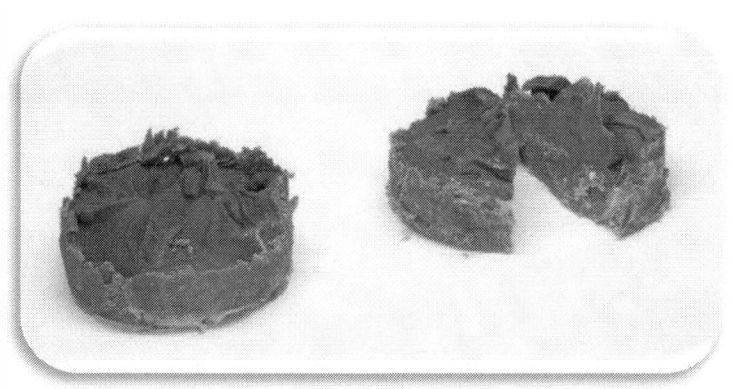

Instructions:

1. Combine all ingredients in a cup or small bowl. Mix well.
2. Freeze for about 2 hours. Serve or store in a container in the fridge.

White Chocolate Fat Bombs

Prep time: 15 min (+ 1 hr)

Cooking time: 0 min

Servings: 8

Nutrients per serving:

Total Carbs – 0 g

Net Carbs – 0 g

Fat – 10 g

Protein – 0 g

Calories – 125

Ingredients:

- ¼ cup cocoa butter
- ¼ cup coconut oil
- 10 drops vanilla flavored stevia

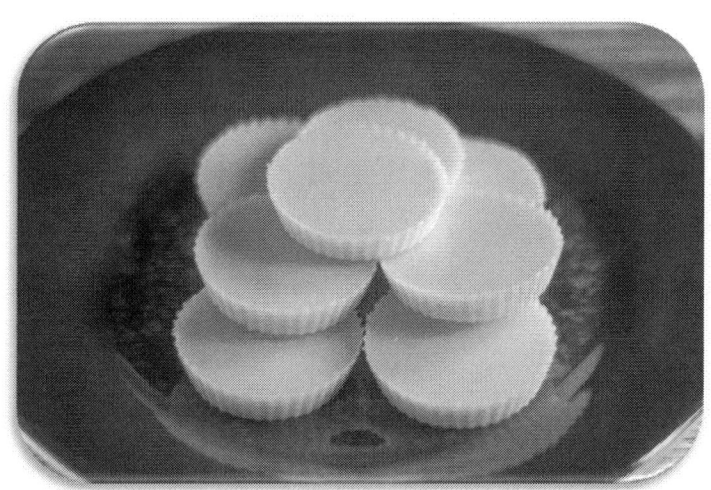

Instructions:

1. Melt together cocoa butter and coconut oil over low heat.
2. Add vanilla flavored stevia drops.
3. Fill 8 molds with the mixture. Let chill for 1 hour.
4. Remove from molds. Serve, or store in the fridge.

Low Carb Red Velvet Fat Bombs

Prep time: 15 min (+ 40 min)

Cooking time: 0 min

Servings: 24

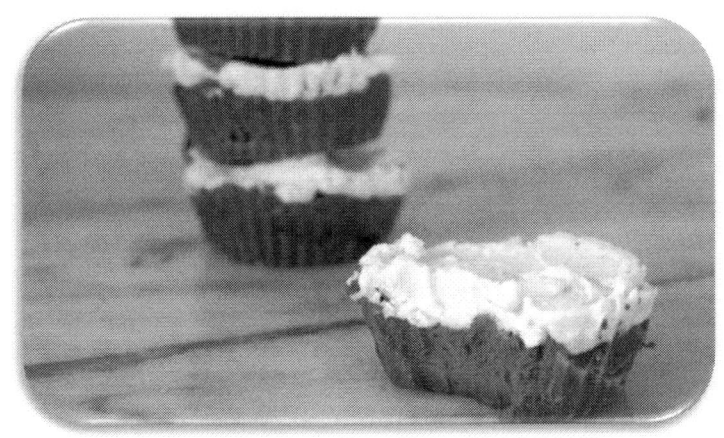

Nutrients per serving:

Total Carbs – 2 g

Net Carbs – 1.2 g

Fat – 9 g

Protein – 1 g

Calories – 85

Ingredients:

- 3.5 oz 90% dark chocolate
- 4.5 oz cream cheese, softened
- 3.5 oz butter, softened
- 3 tbsp Natvia
- 1 tsp vanilla extract
- 4 drops red food coloring
- 1/3 cup heavy cream, whipped

Instructions:

1. In a heatproof bowl, melt the chocolate in a microwave.
2. Combine the remaining ingredients, except the whipped cream, with a hand mixer.
3. Add the melted chocolate and mix for 2 minutes.
4. Fill a piping bag with the mixture and transfer the fat bomb mixture into a lined tray. Refrigerate for 40 minutes.
5. Top with whipped cream, cut into servings and serve.

Almond Pistachio Fat Bombs

Prep time: 30 min (+ 8 hr)

Cooking time: 0 min

Servings: 36 squares

Nutrients per serving:

Total Carbs – 3.1 g

Net Carbs – 1.2 g

Fat –17.4 g

Protein – 2.2 g

Calories – 170

Ingredients:

- ½ cup cacao butter, melted
- 1 cup all natural roasted almond butter
- 1 cup creamy coconut butter
- 1 cup coconut oil, firm
- ½ cup full-fat coconut milk
- ¼ cup ghee
- 1 tbsp pure vanilla extract
- 2 tsp chai spice
- ¼ tsp pure almond extract
- ¼ tsp Himalayan salt
- ¼ cup raw shelled pistachios, chopped

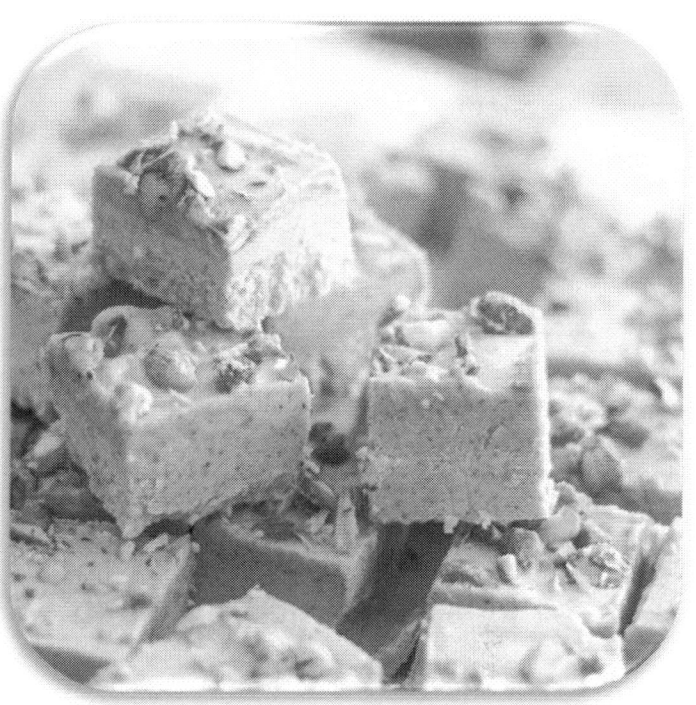

Instructions:

1. Microwave the cacao butter until melted.
2. Combine all the ingredient except the cacao butter and pistachios. Mix with a hand mixer.
3. Pour the melted cacao butter right into the almond mixture, mix well.
4. Transfer the mixture to a baking pan, sprinkle with pistachios. Refrigerate overnight.
5. Cut into 36 squares and serve.

Espresso Fat Bombs

Prep time: 20 min (+ 4 hr)

Cooking time: 0 min

Servings: 24

Nutrients per serving:

Total Carbs – 1.3 g

Net Carbs – 0.3 g

Fat – 6.8 g

Protein – 0.3 g

Calories – 63

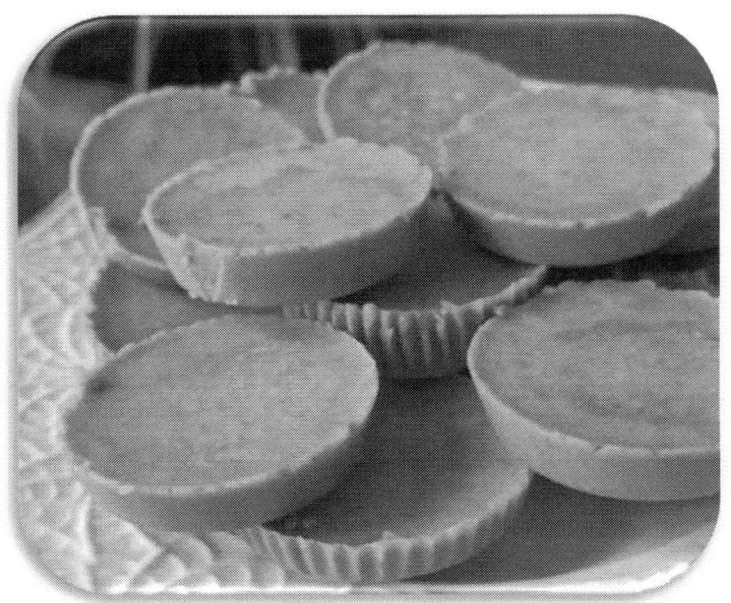

Ingredients:

- 5 tbsp unsalted Kerrygold butter, softened
- 3 oz cream cheese softened
- 2 oz espresso
- 4 tbsp coconut oil
- 2 tbsp heavy whipping cream
- 2 tbsp monk fruit sweetener

Instructions:

1. Melt together all ingredients except the sweetener in a double boiler for 3-4 min.
2. Add the sweetener. Mix all ingredients with a hand-mixer.
3. Spoon the mixture into silicone muffin molds. Freeze for 4 hours.
4. Remove fat bombs from the silicone molds. Serve.

Peanut Butter Chocolate Chip Fat Bombs

Prep time: 10 min (+ 4 hr)

Cooking time: 0 min

Servings: 24

Nutrients per serving:

Total Carbs – 3.5 g

Net Carbs – 1.2 g

Fat – 6 g

Protein – 1.5 g

Calories – 63

Ingredients:

- 1 package (8 oz) cream cheese
- 6-8 tbsp peanut butter
- 2 tbsp grass-fed butter
- 1 tbsp vanilla
- 1-2 tbsp xylitol
- 1 (9 oz) package dark chocolate chips

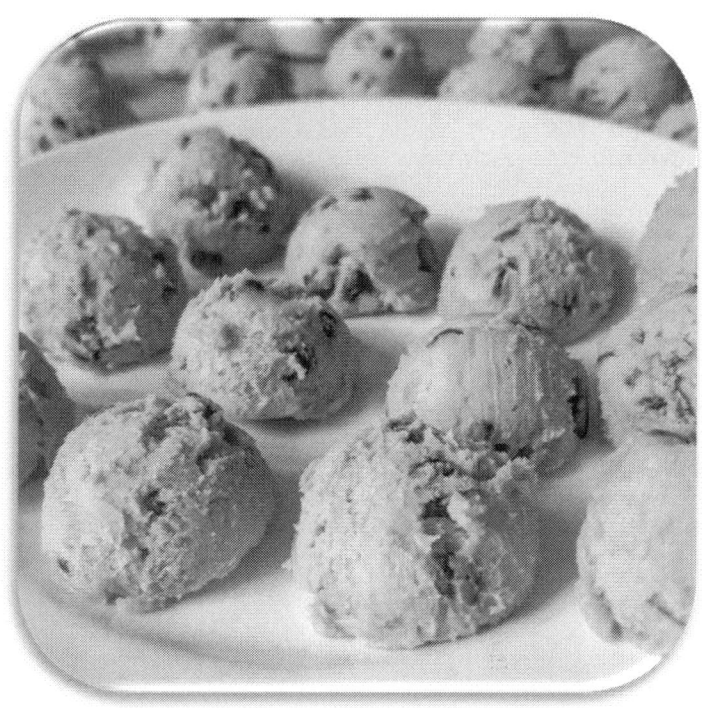

Instructions:

1. Mix all ingredients except the chocolate chips with a hand mixer.
2. Stir in chocolate chips.
3. Place the mixture in silicone candy molds. Freeze for 4 hours. Serve.

Coconut & Almond Fat Bombs

Prep time: 25 min (+ 40 min)

Cooking time: 5 min

Servings: 15

Nutrients per serving:

Total Carbs – 1.9g

Net Carbs – 0.5 g

Fat – 13 g

Protein – 3 g

Calories – 136

Ingredients:

- 1.7 oz unsalted butter
- 14 oz ricotta
- 20 drops stevia
- 1 tbsp psyllium husk
- 1/3 cup coconut, shredded
- ¾ tsp cardamom
- ½ tsp vanilla extract, unsweetened
- 2 tbsp coconut oil
- 2/3 cup almonds

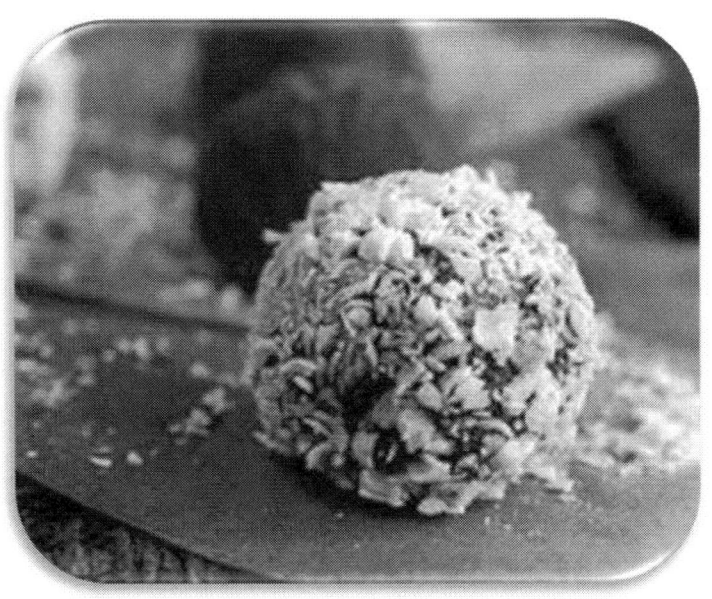

Instructions:

1. Melt butter in a saucepan, then mix in the ricotta.
2. Combine all the ingredients except the almonds and shredded coconut. Add the mixture to the melted cheese mixture. Cool.
3. Roll the mixture into balls, and press an almond inside of each.
4. Roll the balls in shredded coconut to coat. Refrigirate for 30 min. Serve.

Perfect Keto Peaches & Cream Fat Bombs

Prep time: 10 min (+ 4 hr)

Cooking time: 0 min

Servings: 24

Nutrients per serving:

Total Carbs – 1 g

Net Carbs – 0.9 g

Fat –4.2 g

Protein – 0.5 g

Calories – 43

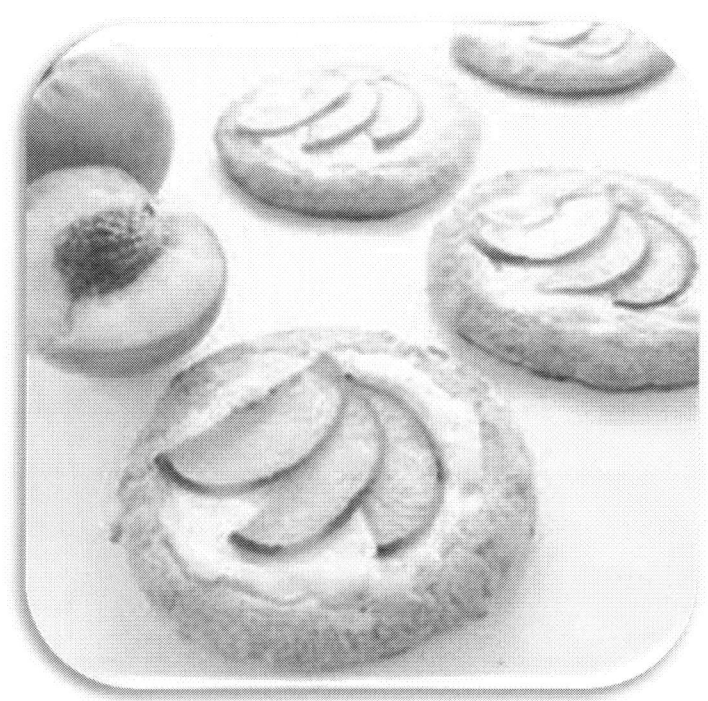

Ingredients:

- 4 tbsp unsalted Kerrygold butter, softened
- 6 oz cream cheese, softened
- 1 cup frozen peaches, slightly warmed
- 2 tsp Perfect Keto Peaches & Cream Ketone Supplement
- 3 ½ tbsp monk fruit sweetener, divided

Instructions:

1. In a medium-sized bowl, combine all ingredients except half of the sweetener with a hand mixer.
2. Spoon the mixture into silicone molds. Top each bomb with remaining sweetener.
3. Freeze for 4 hours.
4. Remove fat bombs from silicone molds and serve.

Pumpkin Spice Fat Bombs

Prep time: 10 min (+ 4 hr)

Cooking time: 10 min

Servings: 24

Nutrients per serving:

Total Carbs – 3.1 g

Net Carbs – 1 g

Fat – 8.2 g

Protein – 0.7 g

Calories – 78

Ingredients:

- ½ cup pecans
- ½ cup coconut oil
- 4 oz cream cheese, softened
- ½ cup pumpkin purée
- ¼ cup monk fruit sweetener
- 2 tsp pumpkin pie spice
- ¼ tsp cinnamon

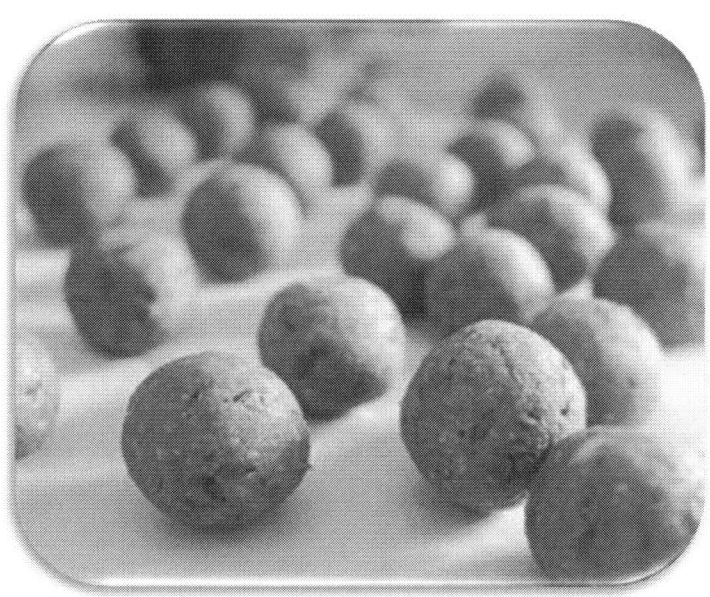

Instructions:

1. In a pan, toast pecans until fragrant.
2. Melt coconut oil and cream cheese over medium-low heat until combined.
3. Mix all ingredients in a bowl.
4. Spoon the mixture into silicone molds, top with toasted pecans, and sprinkle with cinnamon.
5. Freeze for 4 hours. Serve.

Baked Brie with Almonds

Prep time: 10 minutes

Cooking time: 15 minutes

Servings: 8

Nutrition facts per serving:

Total carbs – 8 g

Protein – 8.4 g

Total fat – 12 g

Calories – 187

Ingredients:

- 14 oz round Brie cheese
- ½ cup almonds, toasted
- 6 fresh figs
- 1 Tbsp liquid stevia
- 2 Tbsp water

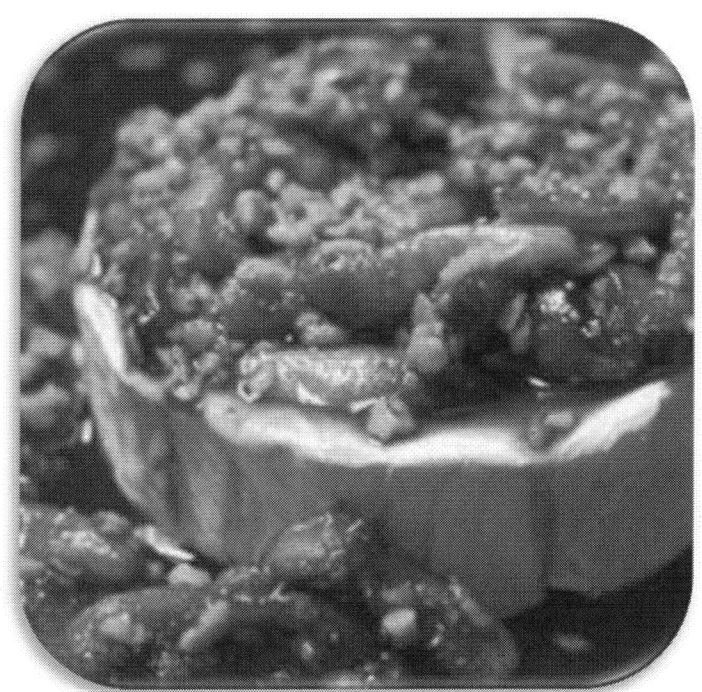

Instructions:

1. In a saucepan heat water with stevia and add figs. Cook about 10 minutes until soft.
2. Stir in almonds.
3. Place the Brie cheese into a baking dish and pour over the sweet almond mixture.
4. Bake for 15 minutes at 325°F.

Berries & Cream Fat Bombs

Prep time: 5 min (+ 8 hr)

Cooking time: 0 min

Servings: 24

Nutrients per serving:

Total Carbs – 2.9 g

Net Carbs – 1.4 g

Fat –5.9 g

Protein – 0.8 g

Calories – 61

Ingredients:

- 2 cups mixed berries, frozen
- 6 tbsp butter, softened
- 8 oz cream cheese, softened
- 2 tbsp golden monk fruit sweetener
- 1 tsp vanilla extract

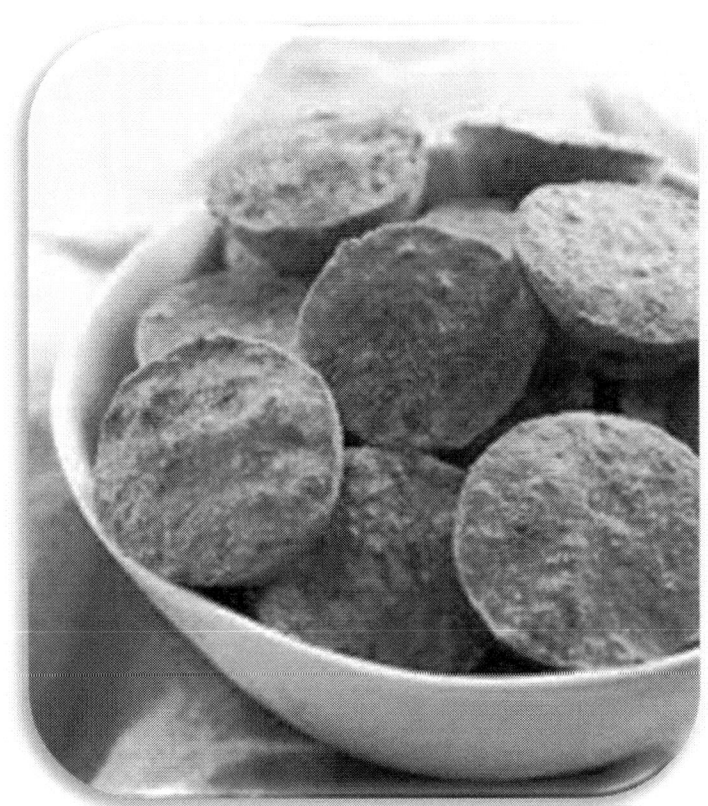

Instructions:

1. Microwave frozen berries until thawed, about 1 minute.
2. Blend all ingredients in a food processor.
3. Spoon mixture into silicone molds and freeze for overnight.
4. Pop fat bombs out of molds and serve.

Blueberry Bliss Fat Bombs

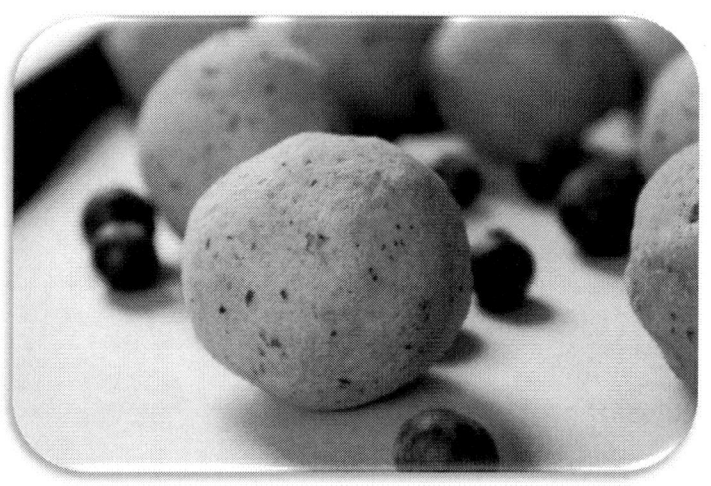

Prep time: 10 min (+ 1 hr)

Cooking time: 0 min

Servings: 30

Nutrients per serving:

Total Carbs – 6.1 g

Net Carbs – 1.4 g

Fat – 14.4 g

Protein –2.2 g

Calories – 161

Ingredients:

- 2 cups raw cashews, soaked in water for 2 hours
- 14 oz frozen blueberries
- 1 cup coconut oil
- ½ cup coconut butter
- ¼–½ tsp stevia

Instructions:

1. Microwave blueberries for about 1 minute, until slightly warmed.
2. Combine all ingredients in a food processor and blend until mixed. Place the mixture in a bowl and put it in the freezer for 30 minutes.
3. After freezing, form the mixture into small balls.
4. Return balls to freezer for 30 minutes. Serve.

Key Lime Pie Fat Bombs

Prep time: 10 min (+ 1 hr)

Cooking time: 0 min

Servings: 30

Nutrients per serving:

Total Carbs – 4.1 g

Net Carbs – 0.9 g

Fat – 14.7 g

Protein – 2.1 g

Calories – 153

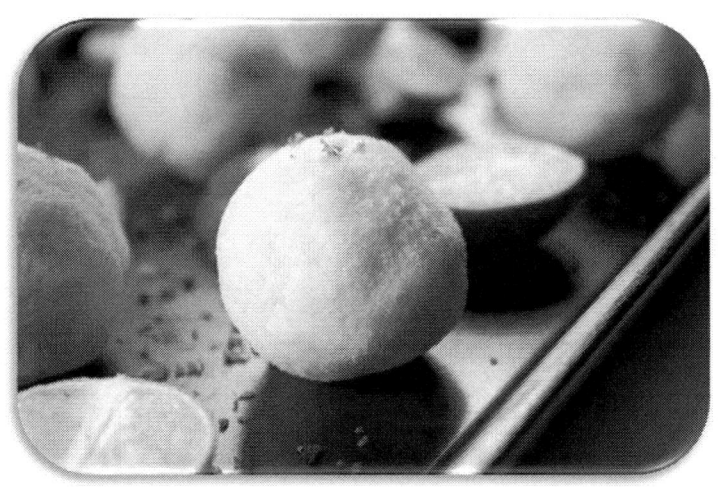

Ingredients:

- 2 cups raw cashews, boiled for 12 minutes or soaked in water for 2 hours
- 1 cup coconut oil, melted
- ½ cup coconut butter
- ¾ cup Key lime juice
- 1/8 tsp – ¼ tsp powdered stevia

Instructions:

1. Blend all ingredients in a food processor.
2. Freeze for 30 minutes in a medium-sized bowl.
3. Remove the mixture from the freezer and form the mixture into small balls.
4. Freeze fat bombs for 20 minutes. Serve or store refrigerated in a container for up to 1 week.

PBJ Fat Bomb

Prep time: 10 min (+ 1 hr)

Cooking time: 0 min

Servings: 30

Nutrients per serving:

Total Carbs – 3.8 g

Net Carbs – 2 g

Fat –7.3 g

Protein – 2.3 g

Calories – 86

Ingredients:

- ¼ cup + 1 tbsp coconut oil
- 2 cups frozen raspberries
- ¾ cup peanut butter
- ¼ cup coconut flour
- 1/8 tsp–¼ tsp powdered stevia

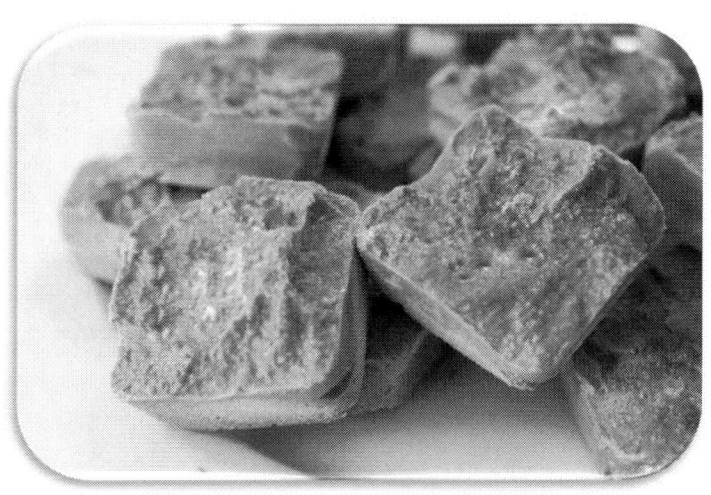

Instructions:

1. Microwave frozen raspberries for about 1 minute, until slightly warmed.
2. Blend all ingredients in a food processor.
3. Spoon mixture into silicone molds and freeze for 1 hour.
4. Remove from freezer, pop fat bombs out of molds. Serve.

Dark Chocolate & Nut Fat Bombs

Prep time: 5 min (+ 2 hr)

Cooking time: 0 min

Servings: 16

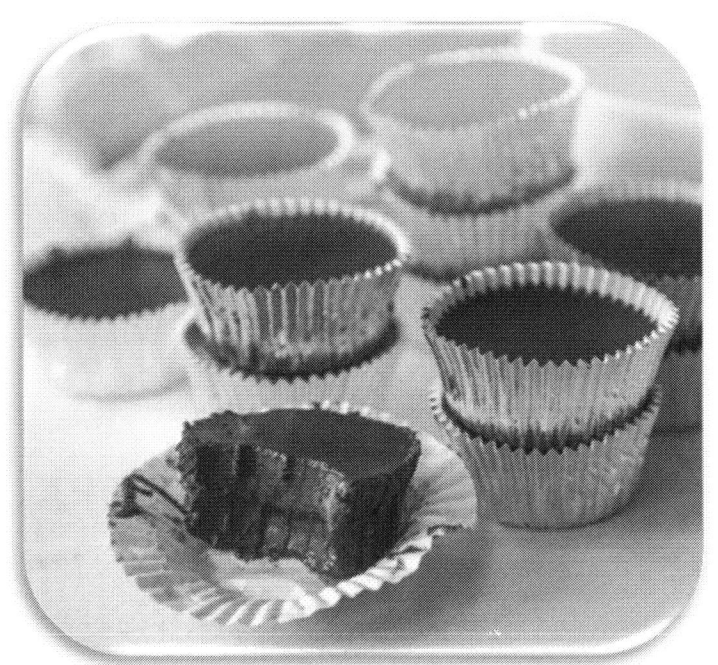

Nutrients per serving:

Total Carbs – 2.8 g

Net Carbs – 1.8 g

Fat – 12 g

Protein – 1.2 g

Calories – 118

Ingredients:

- 4 oz dark chocolate (85% cacao)
- 1 oz extra-virgin coconut oil
- 1 tsp vanilla powder
- 2 tbsp Swerve, powdered
- 1/3 cup cocoa butter
- 2 oz butter, ghee or coconut oil
- 20 drops liquid stevia extract

Instructions:

1. In a double boiler, melt the dark chocolate and cocoa butter.
2. Add the remaining ingredients. Mix well.
3. Pour 2 tbsp of the chocolate mixture into mini-muffin forms or an ice cube tray.
4. Refrigerate for 30 minutes. Serve.

Quick Orange Fat Bombs

Prep time: 10 min (+ 1 hr)

Cooking time: 0 min

Servings: 16

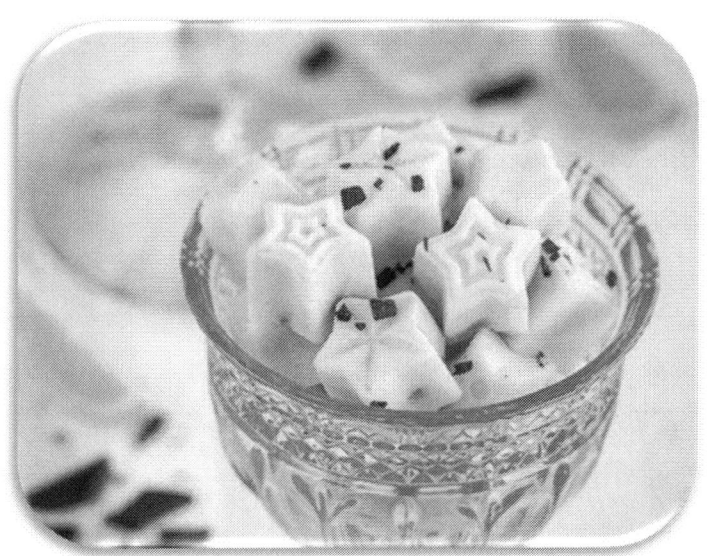

Nutrients per serving:

Total Carbs – 3.2 g

Net Carbs – 1.2 g

Fat –12.8 g

Protein –1 g

Calories – 123

Ingredients:

- 7 oz coconut butter
- ¼ cup coconut oil
- 1 tbsp orange zest, freshly grated
- 2 tbsp erythritol or Swerve, powdered
- 2 tbsp cacao nibs
- Liquid stevia, to taste

Instructions:

1. In a double boiler, melt the coconut butter and coconut oil
2. Add the remaining ingredients except for cacao nibs. Mix well.
3. Fill each mini-muffin cup with 1 tbsp of mixture. Top with the cacao nibs. Refrigerate for 1 hour. Serve.

Raspberry, Chocolate & Coconut Bark

Prep time: 10 min (+ 1 hr)

Cooking time: 8 min

Servings: 16

Nutrients per serving:

Total Carbs – 7.6 g

Net Carbs – 2.7 g

Fat –25.4 g

Protein –2.4 g

Calories – 248

Ingredients:

- 1/3 cup unsweetened flaked coconut
- ½ cup macadamia nuts
- 1 cup coconut butter
- ¼ cup coconut oil
- ¼ cup unsalted butter
- 1/3 cup cocoa powder, unsweetened
- ¼ cup powdered erythritol
- ½ cup raspberries
- Sea salt to taste

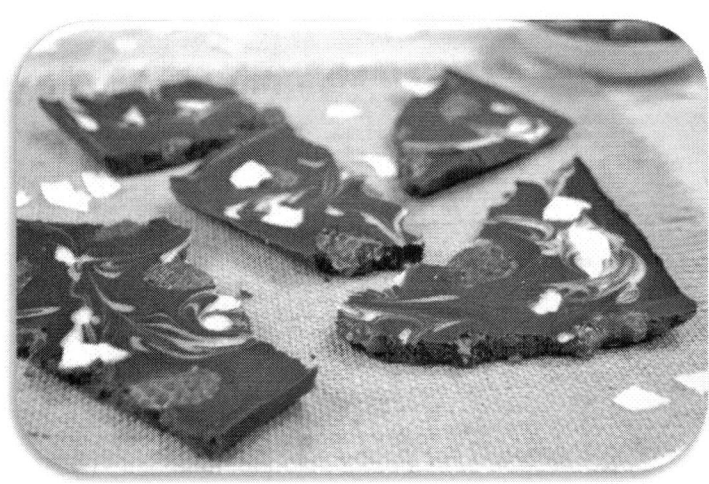

Instructions:

1. Prcheat the oven to 350°F. Toast the coconut flakes and macadamia nuts on a baking sheet for 8 minutes until golden.
2. Melt the coconut butter and coconut oil in a double boiler. Mix in the cocoa powder and erythritol.
3. Pour the chocolate-coconut mixture onto a medium plate. Scatter the raspberries, toasted macadamia nuts and coconut over the chocolate. Sprinkle with the sea salt.
4. Refrigerate for 1 hour. Break into the bark and Serve.

White Chocolate & Raspberry Bark

Prep time: 10 min (+ 1 hr)

Cooking time: 8 min

Servings: 16

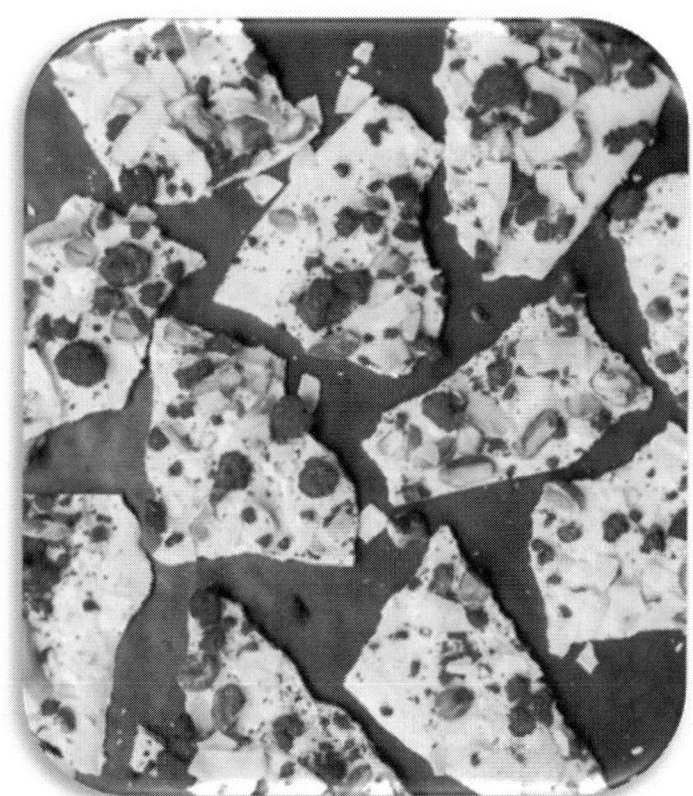

Nutrients per serving:

Total Carbs – 3.2 g

Net Carbs – 2.3 g

Fat – 18 g

Protein – 1.5 g

Calories – 175

Ingredients:

- ½ cup almonds
- 9 oz white chocolate
- 1/3 cup coconut oil
- 2 tsp lemon zest, grated
- 1/3 cup raspberries, frozen

Instructions:

1. Preheat the oven to 350°F. Toast the almonds on a baking sheet for 8 minutes.
2. Melt white chocolate in a double boiler. Mix in the lemon zest. Set aside to cool.
3. Pour the mixture into a parchment-lined pan. Top with the toasted almonds and raspberries. Refrigerate 1 hour. Break into the bark and serve.

Mexican Chili-Chocolate Fudge

Prep time: 20 min (+ 2 hours)

Cooking time: 8 min

Servings: 16

Nutrients per serving:

Total Carbs – 4.1 g

Net Carbs – 1.6 g

Fat –13.2 g

Protein – 1.3 g

Calories – 132

Ingredients:

- 4.5 oz dark chocolate
- ¼ cup strong brewed coffee
- ½ cup unsweetened cocoa powder
- ¼ cup + 1 tbsp powdered erythritol or Swerve
- 1 tsp sugar-free vanilla extract
- ½ tsp cayenne pepper
- ½ cup unsalted butter
- Salt to taste
- 2 avocados, pitted

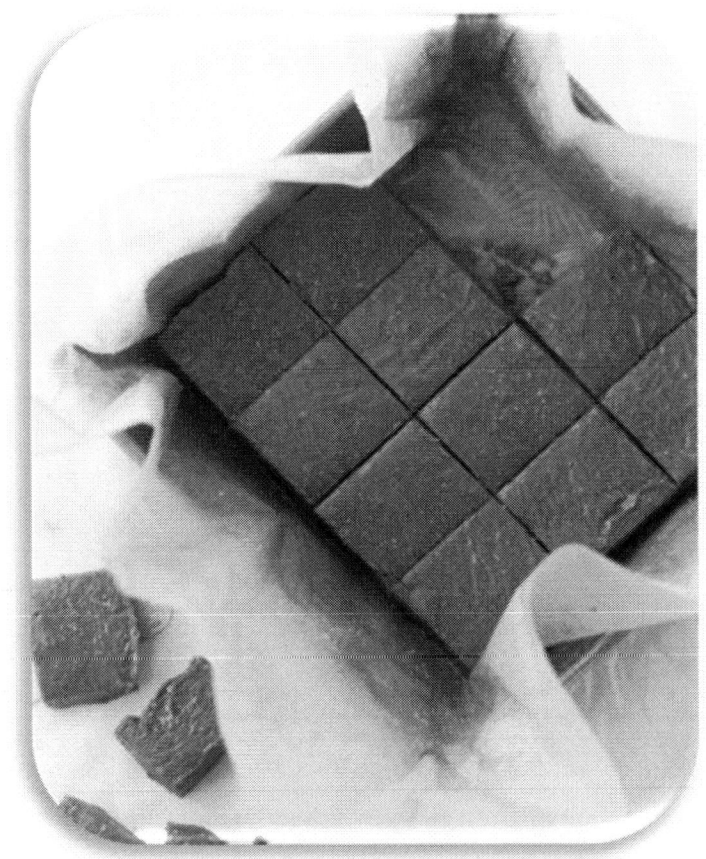

Instructions:

1. In a double boiler melt the dark chocolate. Slowly stir in the coffee. Add the remaining ingredients except for the avocados.
2. Scoop the avocado flesh into a food processor and pulse until smooth. With the processor running, add the chocolate mixture.
3. Spread the batter evenly into a parchment-lined pan with a spatula. Refrigerate for 2 hours or until set. Cut into squares and serve.

Pistachio-Coconut Squares

Prep time: 20 min (+ 1 hr)

Cooking time: 8 min

Servings: 16

Nutrients per serving:

Total Carbs – 8.8 g

Net Carbs – 3..8 g

Fat – 23.9 g

Protein – 4.8 g

Calories – 257

Ingredients:

- 1 cup coconut butter at room temperature
- ¼ cup coconut oil at room temperature
- 2 tbsp powdered erythritol or Swerve
- 2 tsp sugar-free vanilla extract
- 11.5 oz pistachio-coconut butter at room temperature
- ½ cup unsalted pistachio nuts, raw or roasted
- Few drops liquid stevia, to taste

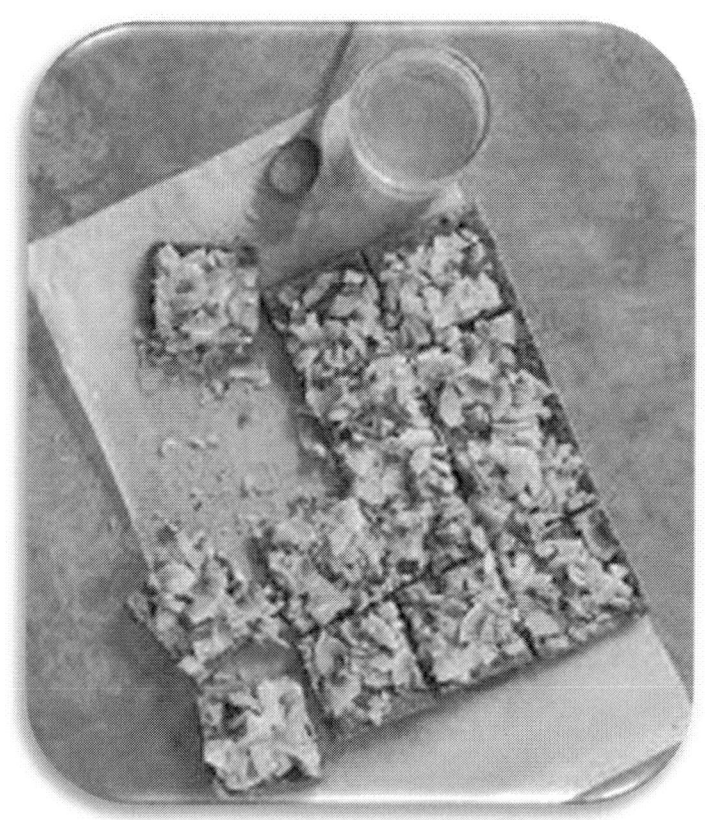

Instructions:

1. Combine the first four ingredients in a mixing bowl. Add the stevia and mix again.
2. Transfer the mixture to a parchment-lined pan or a silicone pan. Spread it evenly into the pan with a spatula.
3. Top with the pistachio-coconut butter and sprinkle with the pistachios. Refrigerate for 1 hour. Cut into squares and serve.

Lemon & Green Tea Cups

Prep time: 15 min (+ 1 hr)

Cooking time: 8 min

Servings: 10

Nutrients per serving:

Total Carbs – 4.2 g

Net Carbs – 1.4 g

Fat – 28.2 g

Protein – 1.3 g

Calories – 261

Ingredients:

- ½ cup macadamia nuts
- ½ cup coconut butter
- ½ cup cacao butter
- ¼ cup coconut oil
- ¼ cup powdered erythritol or Swerve
- Stevia to taste
- 1 tsp matcha green tea powder
- 1 tbsp freshly grated lemon zest

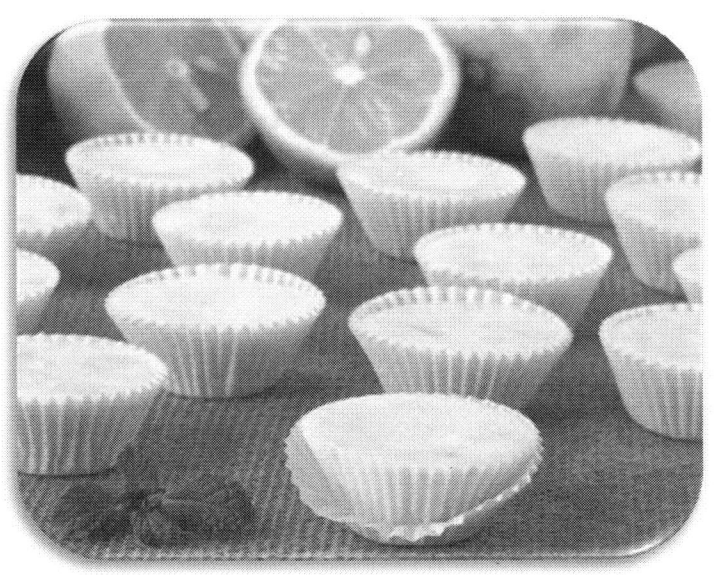

Instructions:

1. In a food processor, combine the first six ingredients. Pulse for 1 minute.
2. Halve the mixture between 2 bowls. Add the matcha powder to one bowl and the lemon zest to the other.
3. Place 10 small paper muffin cups on a tray. Fill each with about 1½ tbsp of the matcha mixture. Top with another 1½ tbsp of the lemon mixture. Refrigerate for 1 hour. Serve.

Chocolate-Avocado Truffles

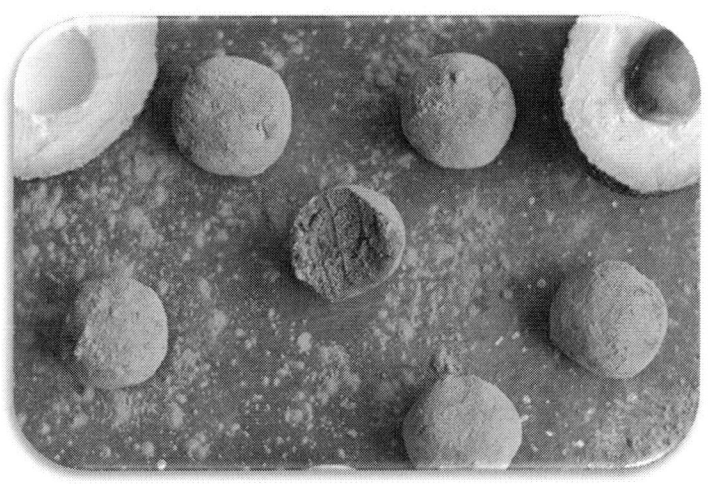

Prep time: 20 min (+ 1 hr 15 min)

Cooking time: 0 min

Servings: 10

Nutrients per serving:

Total Carbs – 5.3 g

Net Carbs – 2.3 g

Fat –12.7 g

Protein – 1.9 g

Calories – 129

Ingredients:

- 3.5 oz dark chocolate
- 1 avocado, peeled and pitted
- ¼ cup coconut butter
- 1 tsp sugar-free vanilla extract
- ½ tsp ground cinnamon
- Salt, stevia to taste
- 2 tbsp cocoa powder

Instructions:

1. Melt the dark chocolate in a double boiler.
2. In a food processor, combine the next five ingredients. Pulse until smooth. Slowly add the melted chocolate. Refrigerate in a bowl for 1 hour.
3. Scoop 10 balls out of the mixture. Coat them in cocoa powder. Refrigerate for 15 minutes. Serve.

Keto Macaroon Fat Bombs

Prep time: 15 min

Cooking time: 15 min

Servings: 10

Nutrients per serving:

Total Carbs – 0.5 g

Net Carbs – 0 g

Fat – 5 g

Protein – 1.8 g

Calories – 46

Ingredients:

- ¼ cup organic almond flour
- ½ cup coconut, shredded
- 2 tbsp Swerve
- 1 tbsp vanilla extract
- 1 tbsp coconut oil
- 3 egg whites

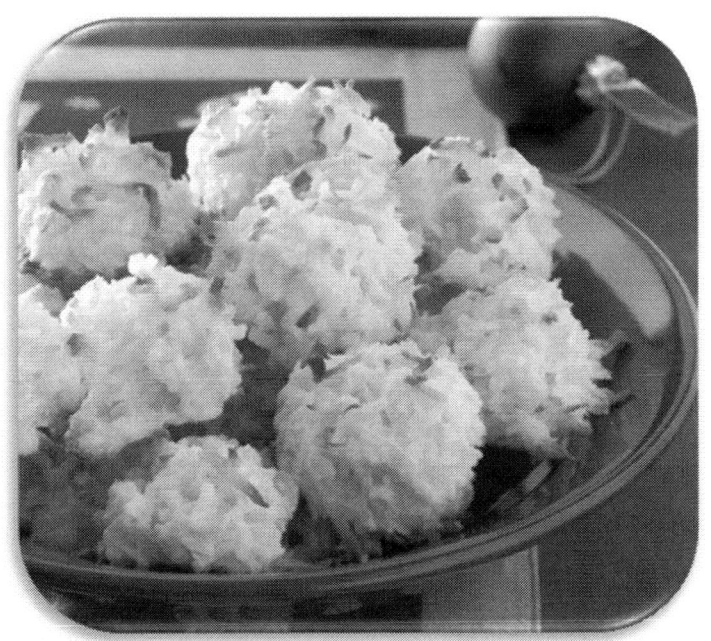

Instructions:

1. Blend the first three ingredients.
2. In a small saucepan, melt the coconut oil, add the vanilla extract.
3. Mix together the melted coconut oil and almond flour mixture.
4. Whisk the egg whites. Fold them into the flour mix.
5. Form the mixture into balls. Serve. Spoon the mixture onto a cookie sheet.
6. Bake at 350°F for 8 minutes. Remove from oven and let cool. Serve.

Almond Butter Fat Bombs

Prep time: 15 min (+ 30 min)

Cooking time: 0 min

Servings: 1

Nutrients per serving:

Total Carbs – 3.6 g

Net Carbs – 1.4 g

Fat –19.1 g

Protein – 3.2 g

Calories – 189

Ingredients:

- ¼ cup almond butter
- ¼ cup unrefined coconut oil
- 2 tbsp cacao powder
- ¼ cup erythritol

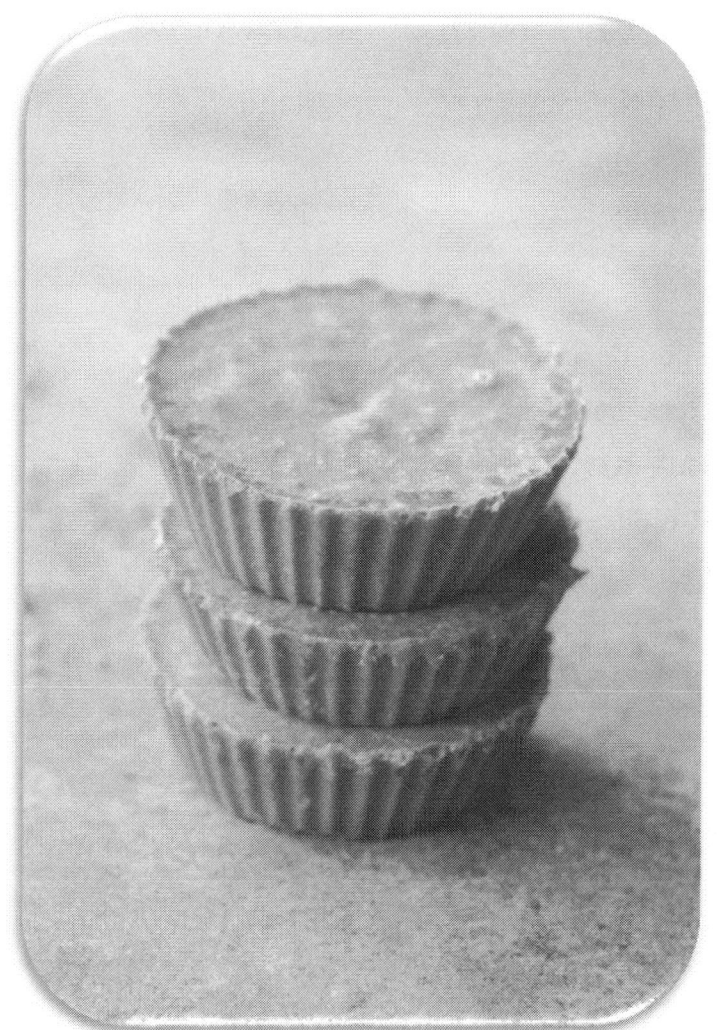

Instructions:

1. Mix together almond butter and coconut oil. Microwave for 30-45 sec or until heated.
2. Add erythritol and cacao powder.
3. Pour into silicone molds. Refrigerate for 30 min. Serve.

Cream Cheese Craters

Prep time: 20 min (+ 2 hr 30 min)

Cooking time: 0 min

Servings: 12

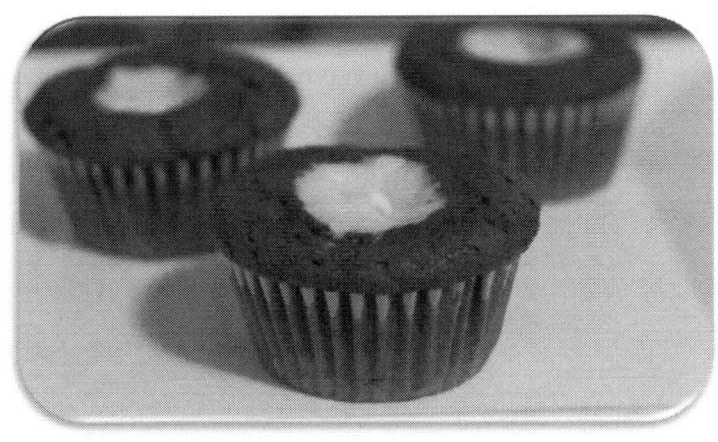

Nutrients per serving:

Total Carbs – 2 g

Net Carbs – 2 g

Fat –10 g

Protein –2 g

Calories – 100

Ingredients:

- ½ cup full-fat cream cheese
- ½ cup walnuts, chopped
- ½ cup grated dark chocolate
- Stevia, to taste

For the filling:

- 4 tbsp grass-fed butter
- 2 tbsp espresso powder
- 2 tbsp heavy cream
- Stevia to taste

Instructions:

1. Mix softened cream cheese, dark chocolate, walnuts, and stevia.
2. Coat the sides of 12 mini-cupcake liners with the mixture to form craters.
3. Freeze for 2 hours.
4. For the filling, melt the butter, and add the remaining ingredients. Stir thoroughly.
5. Add the filling to the craters. Refrigerate for 30 min. Serve.

Bulletproof Fat Bombs

Prep time: 15 min (+ 4 hr)

Cooking time: 0 min

Servings: 20

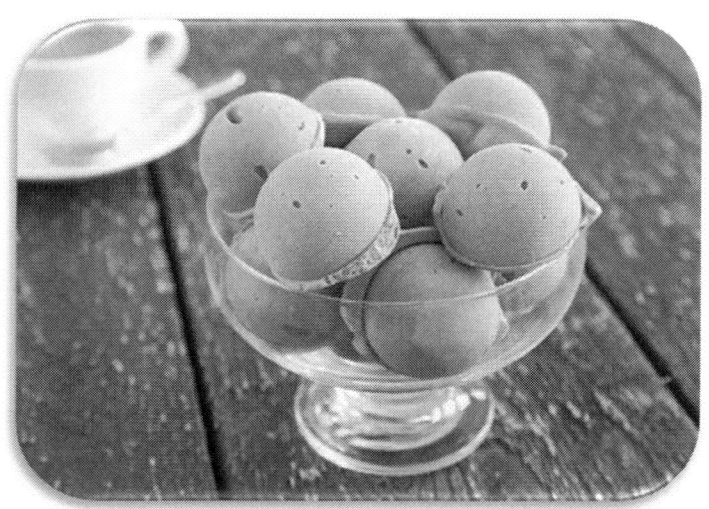

Nutrients per serving:

Total Carbs – 0.7 g

Net Carbs – 0.5 g

Fat –8.1 g

Protein – 0.8 g

Calories – 77

Ingredients:

- 1 cup creamed coconut milk
- ¼ cup butter, grass-fed
- 2 tbsp coconut oil
- 2 tbsp cocoa powder, unsweetened
- ¼ cup powdered erythritol,
- 15 drops stevia extract
- ½ cup strong brewed coffee

Instructions:

1. Combine first four ingredients.
2. Pulse erythritol and stevia in a blender. Pour in the coffee and pulse again.
3. Combine the coconut and coffee mixtures, and pour into an ice cream maker. Process for 30-60 minutes.
4. Spoon 2 tbsp of the ice cream into each compartment of an ice tray.
5. Put in the freezer for 2-3 hours. Serve.

Fudge Fat Bombs

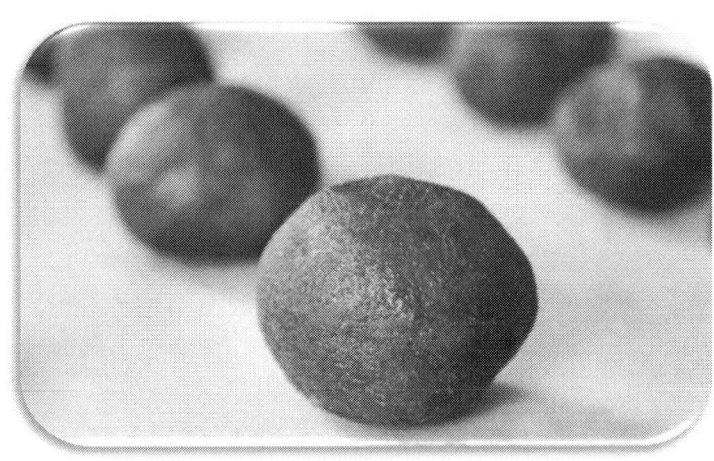

Prep time: 15 min (+ 2 hr)

Cooking time: 0 min

Servings: 30

Nutrients per serving:

Total Carbs – 4.5 g

Net Carbs – 3.6 g

Fat –13.5 g

Protein – 2.4 g

Calories – 144

Ingredients:

- 1 cup almond butter
- 1 cup coconut oil
- ½ cup unsweetened cocoa powder
- 1/3 cup coconut flour
- ¼ tsp powdered stevia
- 1/16 tsp pink Himalayan salt

Instructions:

1. Combine butter and coconut oil and melt over medium heat.
2. Stir in remaining ingredients, mix thoroughly.
3. Pour mixture into silicone molds and put in freezer to solidify for 2 hours. Serve.

Keto Fat Bombs

Over 90 Recipes of Keto Snacks and Treats for Fat Burning and Healthy Weight Loss

Second Edition

Adele Baker

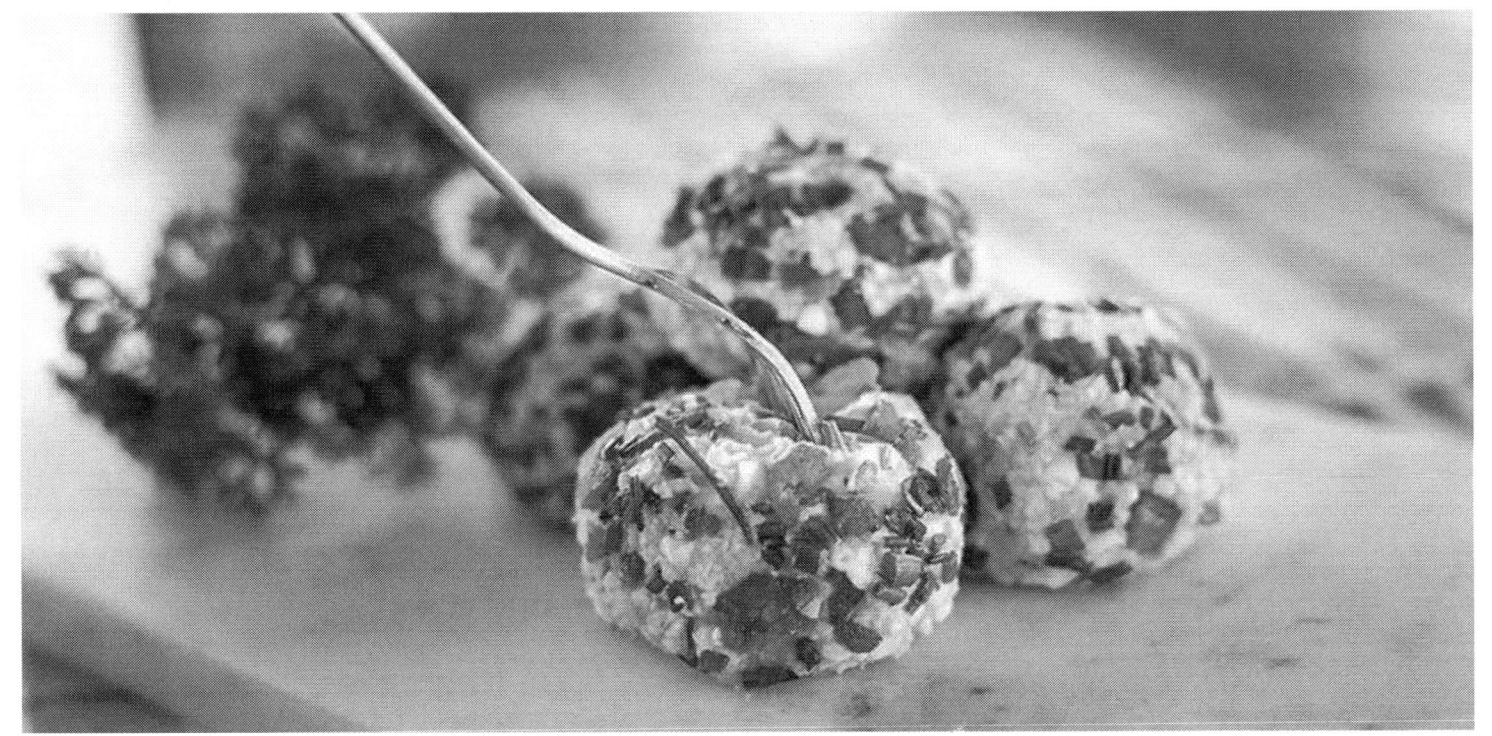

INTRODUCTION

Have you ever wanted to have more energy in your day, feel better, and look better? Many people have found a way to achieve a better life with a simple diet. There is no magic pill; rather, it is as simple as developing an eating plan that gives your body the nutrients it needs.

What is this magic eating plan? It is known as the Ketogenic Diet. While most of us are accustomed to the old food guide pyramids and the newer plate renditions released by health and government institutions, many have become frustrated with a lack of improvement in health despite following these guidelines. If you're looking to lose weight, lower your blood glucose, impact your neurological health, or just feel better overall, the keto diet is sure to help!

Fat bombs are are high fat, low carb snacks that you can use as a quick breakfast, a quick mid-afternoon snack, a pre- or post-workout snack, or as extra fuel during your day. Fat bombs can be savory or sweet, but they are always made from healthy fats and low carb ingredients.

Sweet fat bombs are best at keeping pesky sugar cravings under control, and savory fat bombs will indulge the senses and anchor blood sugars to a steady low number! Some of the fat bombs are really a small meal in themselves, designed to accommodate the demands of busy lifestyles. Sweet fat bombs double as great desserts for family and friends, or healthy snacks for kids. Now everyone can relish the benefits of this way of eating and stay away from highly processed and sugary foods

This book offers over 90 delicious fat bomb recipes that will enable you to stay true to a ketogenic way of life. The fat bomb is truly the secret weapon every healthy eater should have in his or her arsenal to eat clean, stay full, and feel absolutely satisfied instead of deprived. It's time to embrace not only a diet but a new and healthy way of life!

SAVORY FAT BOMBS

Avocado, Macadamia, & Prosciutto Balls

Prep time: 7 minutes

Cooking time: 0 minutes

Servings: 6

Nutrients per serving:

Carbohydrates – 5 g

Net Carbs – 2 g

Fat – 17 g

Protein – 3 g

Calories – 170

Ingredients:

- 4 oz macadamia nuts
- 4 oz avocado pulp
- 1 oz cooked prosciutto, crumbled
- ¼ tsp freshly ground black pepper

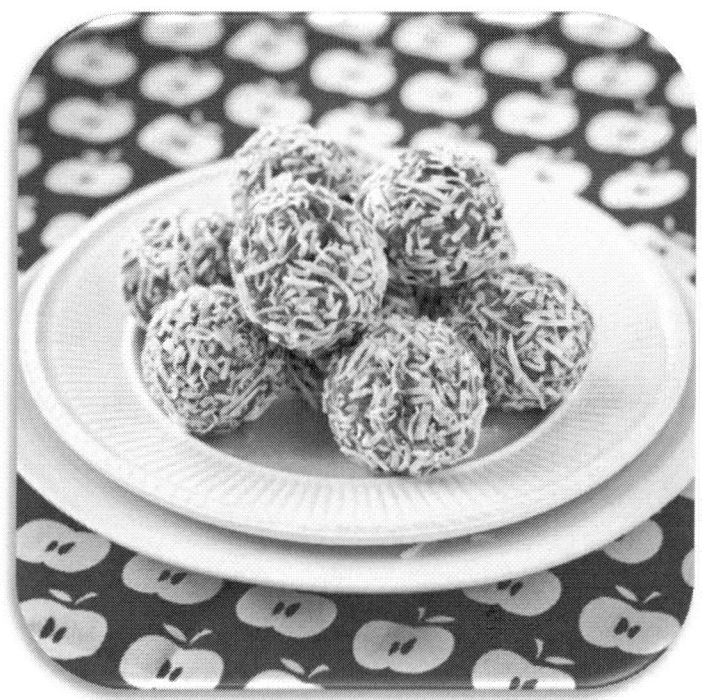

Instructions:

1. In a small food processor, pulse macadamia nuts until evenly crumbled. Divide in half.
2. In a small bowl, combine avocado, half the macadamia nuts, prosciutto crumbles, and pepper. Mix well with a fork.
3. Form mixture into 6 balls.
4. Place remaining crumbled macadamia nuts on a medium plate and roll individual balls through to coat evenly.
5. Serve immediately.

Bacon Jalapeño Balls

Prep time: 10 minutes

Cooking time: 0 minutes

Servings: 6

Nutrients per serving:

Carbohydrates – 1 g

Net Carbs – 0 g

Fat – 11 g

Protein – 7 g

Calories – 135

Ingredients:

- 3 oz bacon, cooked, fat reserved
- 3 oz cream cheese
- 2 Tbsp bacon fat, reserved
- 1 tsp jalapeño pepper, seeded, finely chopped
- 1 Tbsp cilantro, finely chopped

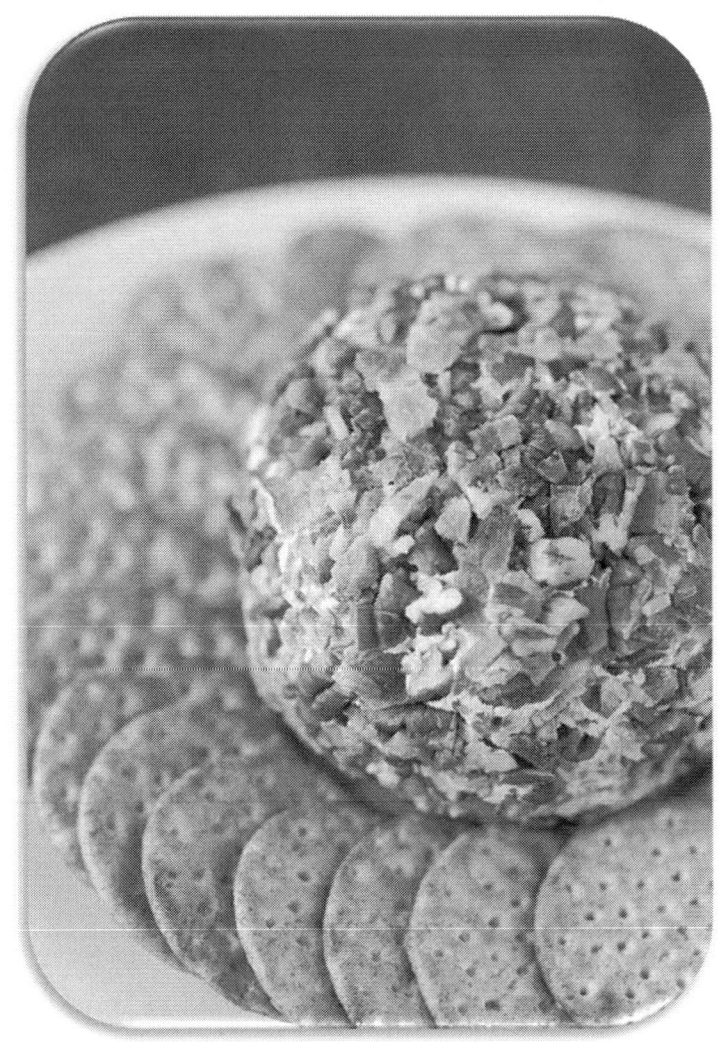

Instructions:

1. On a cutting board, chop bacon into small pieces.
2. In a bowl, combine cream cheese, bacon fat, jalapeño, and cilantro. Mix well with a fork.
3. Form mixture into 6 balls.
4. Place bacon pieces on a medium plate and roll individual balls through to coat evenly.
5. Serve immediately or refrigerate up to 3 days.

Bacon Maple Pancake Balls

Prep time: 10 minutes

Cooking time: 0 minutes

Servings: 6

Nutrients per serving:

Carbohydrates – 1 g

Net Carbs – 0 g

Fat – 13 g

Protein – 6 g

Calories – 148

Ingredients:

- 3 oz bacon, cooked
- 3 oz cream cheese
- ½ tsp maple flavor
- ¼ tsp salt
- 3 Tbsp crushed pecans

Instructions:

1. On a cutting board, chop bacon into small pieces.
2. In a bowl, combine cream cheese and bacon with maple flavor and salt. Mix well with a fork.

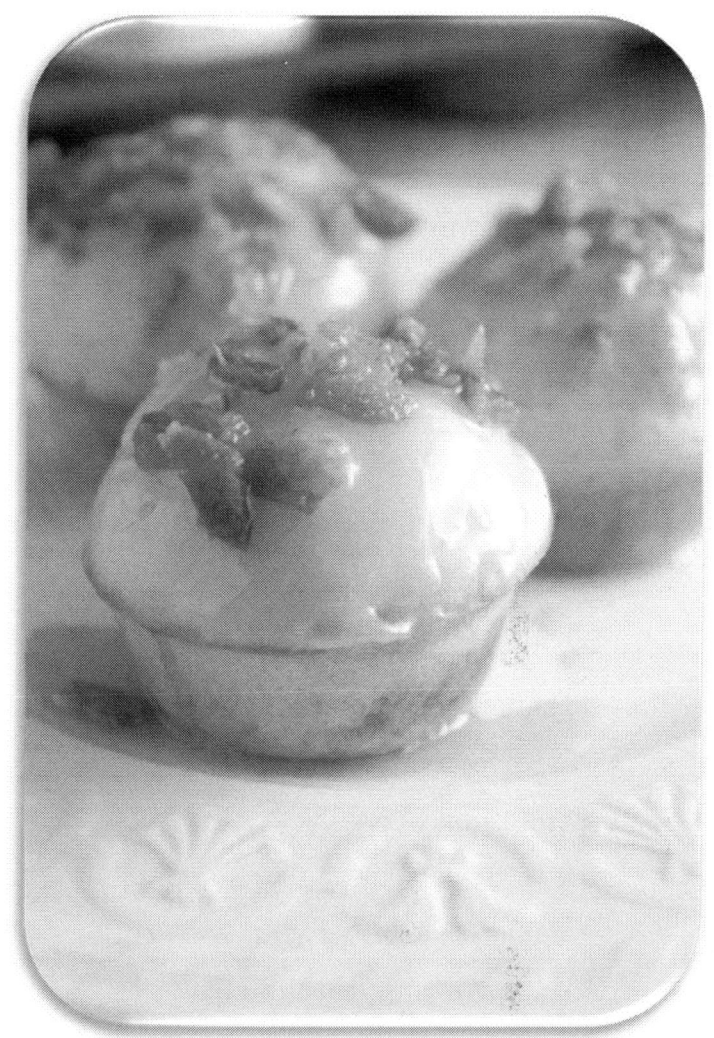

3. Form mixture into 6 balls.
4. Place crushed pecans on a medium plate and roll individual balls through to coat evenly.
5. Serve immediately or refrigerate up to 3 days.

Barbecue Balls

Prep time: 2 hours 5 minutes

Cooking time: 0 minutes

Servings: 6

Nutrients per serving:

Carbohydrates – 1 g

Net Carbs – 0 g

Fat – 13 g

Protein – 3 g

Calories – 154

Ingredients:

- 4 oz cream cheese
- 4 Tbsp bacon fat
- ½ tsp smoke flavor
- 2 drops stevia glycerite
- 1/8 tsp apple cider vinegar
- 1 Tbsp sweet smoked chili powder
- 3 Tbsp barbecue sauce

Instructions:

1. In a food processor, combine all ingredients except chili powder until a smooth, creamy mixture forms, about 30 seconds.

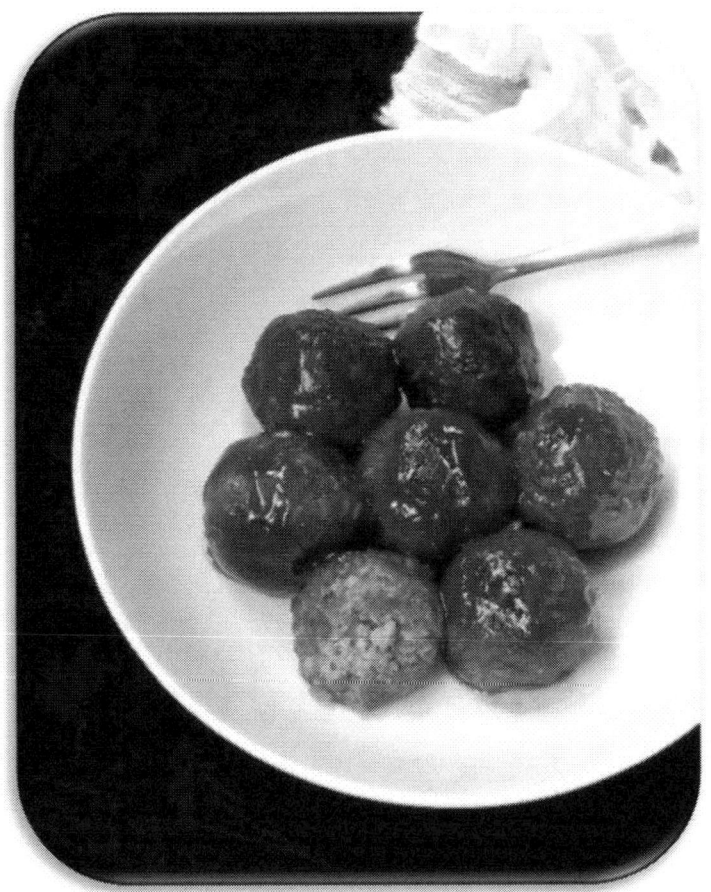

2. Transfer mixture to a small bowl, then refrigerate 2 hours.
3. Form into 6 balls.
4. Sprinkle balls with chili powder, rolling around to coat all sides. Pour barbecue sauce over balls.
5. Serve or refrigerate up to 3 days.

Olive Cheese balls

Prep time: 5 minutes

Cooking time: 15 minutes

Servings: 12

Nutrients per serving:

Total Carbs – 5 g

Fat – 8 g

Protein – 4 g

Calories – 110

Ingredients:

- 24 pimento stuffed olives
- 1 cup Cheddar, shredded
- 2 Tbsp butter, softened
- ½ cup Keto friendly flour (almond/coconut/etc)
- Cayenne pepper to taste

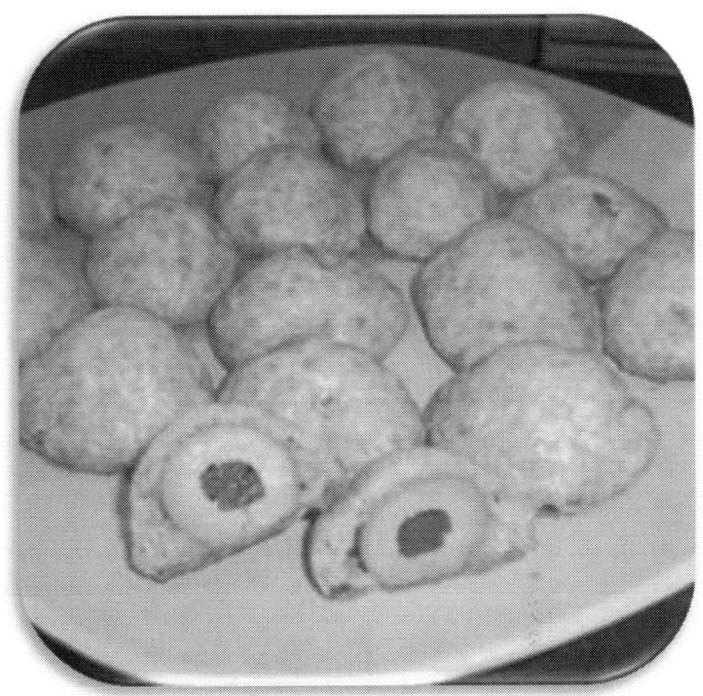

Instructions:

1. In a medium bowl combine cheese and butter, and stir in the flour. Mix to combine and season with pepper.
2. Wrap the cheese, butter and flour mixture around each olive.
3. Arrange the olive cheese balls on a baking sheet lined with parchment paper.
4. Bake for 15 minutes at 400°F.

Kalamata Olive and Feta Balls

Prep time: 2 hours 5 minutes

Cooking time: 0 minutes

Servings: 6

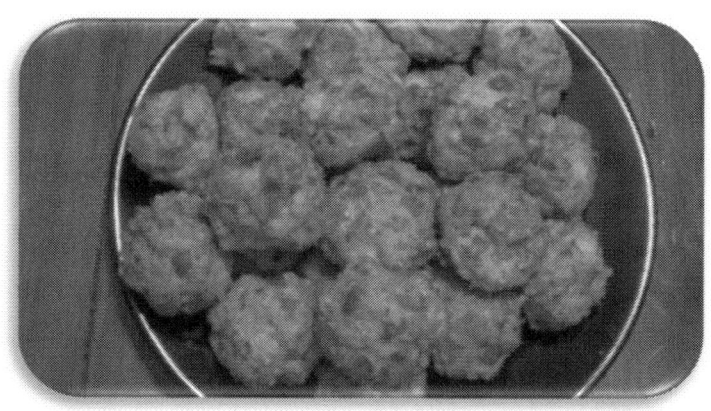

Nutrients per serving:

Carbohydrates – 2 g

Net Carbs – 0 g

Fat – 5 g

Protein – 2 g

Calories – 61

Ingredients:

- 2 oz cream cheese
- 2 oz feta
- 12 large kalamata olives, pitted
- 1/8 tsp fresh thyme,finely chopped
- 1/8 tsp fresh lemon zest

Instructions:

1. In a food processor, combine all ingredients until a coarse, doughy mix is made, about 30 seconds.
2. Transfer the mixture to a small bowl, then refrigerate 2 hours.
3. Form into 6 balls.
4. Serve or refrigerate up to 3 days.

Brie Hazelnut Balls

Prep time: 2 hours 5 minutes

Cooking time: 0 minutes

Servings: 6

Nutrients per serving:

Carbohydrates – 2 g

Net Carbs – 0 g

Fat – 11 g

Protein – 5 g

Calories – 121

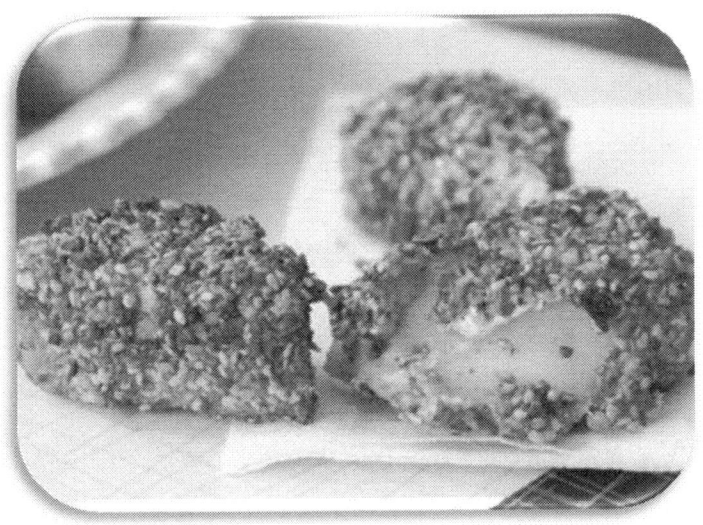

Ingredients:

- 4 oz Brie
- 2 oz hazelnuts, toasted
- 1/8 tsp fresh thyme, finely chopped

Instructions:

1. In a food processor, combine all ingredients until a coarse, doughy mixture is formed, about 30 seconds.
2. Scrape mixture and transfer to a bowl, then refrigerate 2 hours.
3. Form into 6 balls.
4. Serve or refrigerate up to 3 days.

Carbonara Balls

Prep time: 8 minutes

Cooking time: 0 minutes

Servings: 6

Nutrients per serving:

Carbohydrates – 1 g

Net Carbs – 0 g

Fat – 12 g

Protein – 8 g

Calories – 148

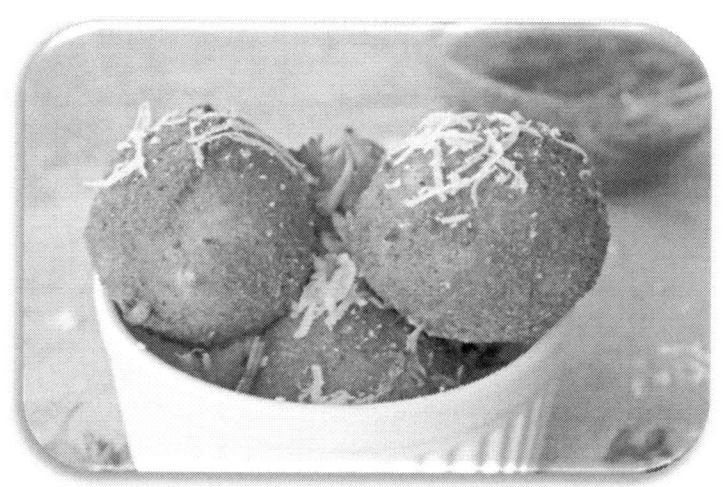

Ingredients:

- 3 oz bacon, cooked
- 3 oz mascarpone
- 2 large hard-boiled egg yolks
- ¼ tsp freshly ground black pepper

Instructions:

1. On a cutting board, chop bacon into small pieces.
2. In a small bowl, combine mascarpone, egg yolks, and pepper. Mix well with a fork.
3. Form mascarpone mixture into 6 balls.
4. Place bacon crumbles on a medium plate and roll individual balls through to coat evenly.
5. Serve immediately or refrigerate up to 3 days.

Creamy & Crunchy Egg Balls

Prep time: 40 minutes

Cooking time: 0 minutes

Servings: 6

Nutrients per serving:

Carbohydrates – 0 g

Net Carbs – 0 g

Fat – 6 g

Protein – 4 g

Calories – 67

Ingredients:

- 2 medium hard-boiled eggs
- 2 Tbsp cream cheese
- 1 Tbsp coconut oil, melted
- 2 slices prosciutto, cooked, crumbled

Instructions:

1. Place eggs, cream cheese, and coconut oil in a food processor and pulse until well mixed.
2. Refrigirate mixture for 30 minutes, or until it solidifies.

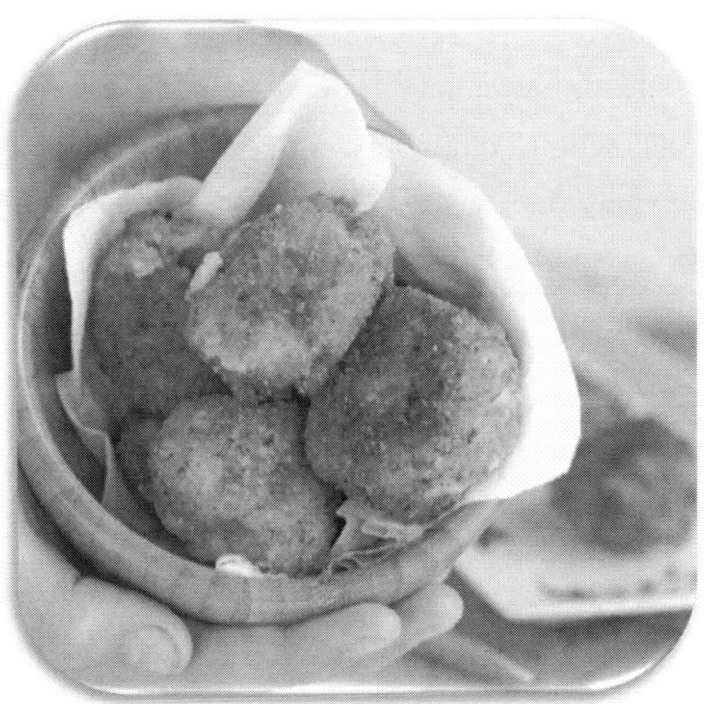

3. Once the egg mixture is solid, remove from refrigerator and shape into 6 balls.
4. Place prosciutto crumbles on a medium plate and roll individual balls through to coat.
5. Serve immediately or refrigerate in an airtight container up to 4 days.

Creamy Olive Balls

Prep time: 40 minutes

Cooking time: 0 minutes

Servings: 6

Nutrients per serving:

Carbohydrates – 6 g

Net Carbs – 2 g

Fat – 4 g

Protein – 3 g

Calories – 71

Ingredients:

- 6 large kalamata olives, pitted
- 2 Tbsp cream cheese
- 1 Tbsp coconut oil, melted
- 2 Tbsp hemp hearts

Instructions:

1. Place olives, cream cheese, and coconut oil in a food processor and pulse until well mixed.
2. Refrigirate mixture for 30 minutes, or until it solidifies.
3. Once the mixture is solid, remove from refrigerator and shape into 6 balls.

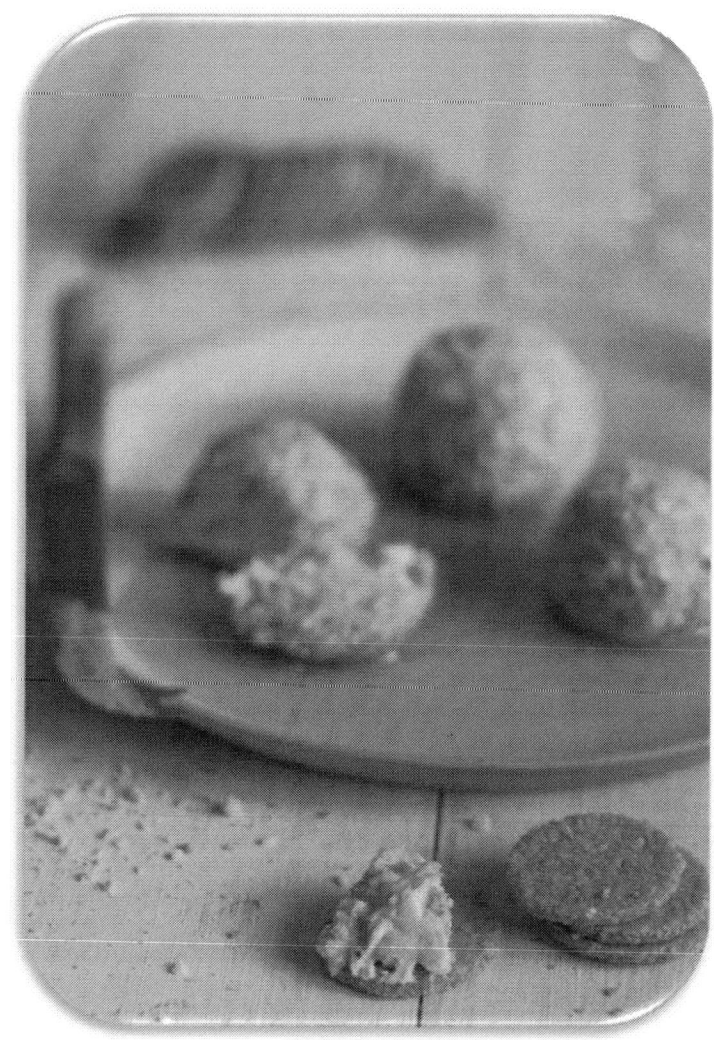

4. Place hemp hearts on a medium plate and roll individual balls through to coat.
5. Serve immediately or refrigerate in an airtight container up to 4 days.

Curried Tuna Balls

Prep time: 10 minutes

Cooking time: 0 minutes

Servings: 6

Nutrients per serving:

Carbohydrates – 1 g

Net Carbs – 0 g

Fat – 8 g

Protein – 5 g

Calories – 93

Ingredients:

- 3 oz tuna in oil, drained
- 2 oz cream cheese
- ¼ tsp curry powder, divided
- 1 oz crumbled macadamia nuts

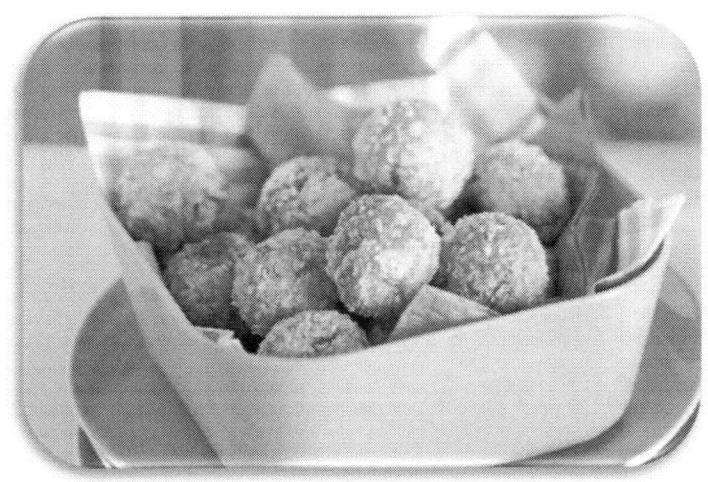

Instructions:

1. In a small food processor, mix tuna, cream cheese, and half the curry powder until smooth, about 30 seconds.
2. Form mixture into 6 balls.
3. Place crumbled macadamia nuts and remaining curry powder on a medium plate and roll individual balls through to coat evenly.
4. Serve or refrigerate up to 3 days.

Egg Tapenade Balls

Prep time: 40 minutes

Cooking time: 0 minutes

Servings: 6

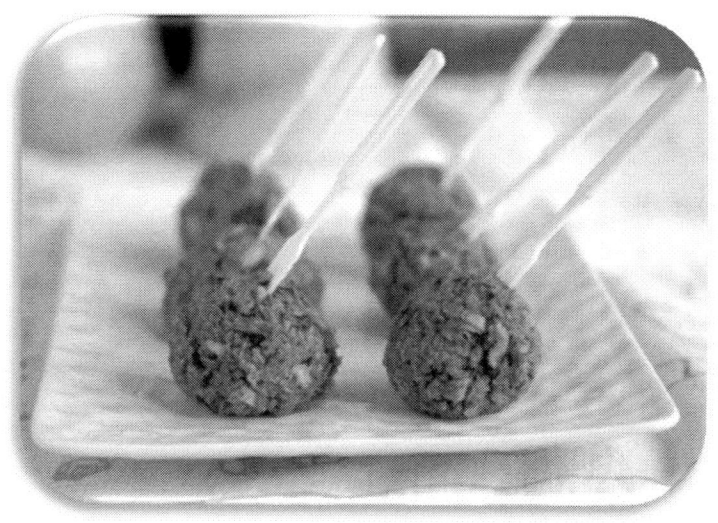

Nutrients per serving:

Carbohydrates – 5 g

Net Carbs – 2 g

Fat – 6 g

Protein – 5 g

Calories – 86

Ingredients:

- 2 large eggs
- 12 large kalamata olives, pitted
- 3 oz anchovy fillet
- 1 Tbsp coconut oil, melted
- 1 Tbsp chia seeds

Instructions:

1. Place eggs, olives, anchovy fillet, and coconut oil in a food processor and pulse until mixed but not over blended.

2. Refrigirate mixture for 30 minutes, or until it solidifies.

3. Once the egg mixture is solid, remove from refrigerator and shape into 6 balls.

4. Place chia seeds on a medium plate and roll individual balls through to coat.

5. Serve immediately or refrigerate in an airtight container up to 4 days.

For the Love of Pork Bombs

Prep time: 1 hour 15 minutes

Cooking time: 10 minutes

Servings: 12

Nutrients per serving:

Carbohydrates – 2 g

Net Carbs – 1 g

Fat – 18 g

Protein – 6 g

Calories – 192

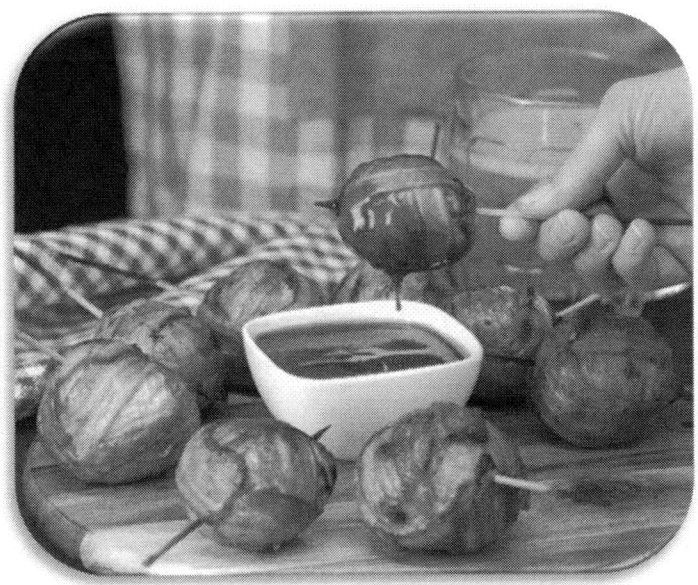

Ingredients:

- 8 slices bacon
- 8 oz Braunschweiger, at room temperature
- ¼ cup pistachio, chopped
- 6 oz cream cheese, at room temperature
- 1 tsp Dijon mustard

Instructions:

1. In a skillet, cook the bacon for 5 minutes per side. Drain on paper towels and let cool. Once cooled, crumble bacon.

2. Place Braunschweiger with pistachios in a small food processor and pulse until just combined.

3. In a small mixing bowl, use a hand blender to whip cream cheese and Dijon mustard until fluffy.

4. Divide meat mixture into 12 equal servings. Roll into balls and cover in a thin layer of cream cheese mixture.

5. Chill at least 1 hour. When ready to serve, place bacon bits on a medium plate, roll balls through to coat evenly, and enjoy.

6. Fat bombs can be refrigerated in an airtight container up to 4 days.

Pizza Balls

Prep time: 8 minutes

Cooking time: 0 minutes

Servings: 6

Nutrients per serving:

Carbohydrates – 1 g

Net Carbs – 0 g

Fat – 8 g

Protein – 3 g

Calories – 82

Ingredients:

- 2 oz fresh mozzarella
- 2 oz cream cheese
- 1 Tbsp olive oil
- 1 tsp tomato paste
- 6 large kalamata olives, pitted
- 12 fresh basil leaves

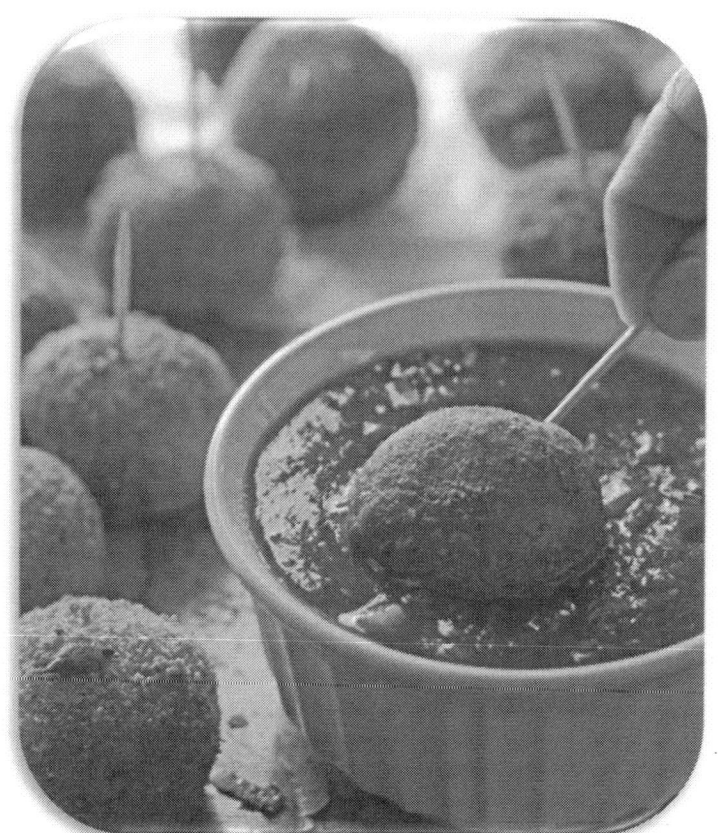

Instructions:

1. In a food processor, mix all ingredients except basil until they form a smooth cream, about 30 seconds.
2. Form mixture into 6 balls.
3. Place 1 basil leaf on top and bottom of each ball and secure with a toothpick.
4. Serve or refrigerate up to 3 days.

Prosciutto and Egg Balls

Prep time: 40 minutes

Cooking time: 0 minutes

Servings: 6

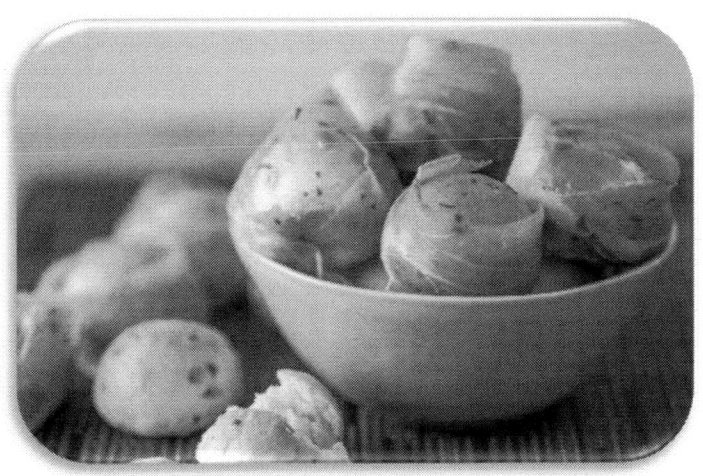

Nutrients per serving:

Carbohydrates – 0 g

Net Carbs – 0 g

Fat – 8 g

Protein – 4 g

Calories – 84

Ingredients:

- 2 medium hard-boiled eggs
- 2 Tbsp mayonnaise
- 1/8 tsp black pepper, freshly ground
- 1/8 tsp sea salt
- 1 Tbsp coconut oil, melted
- 6 slices prosciutto, cooked

Instructions:

1. Place eggs, mayonnaise, pepper, and salt in a small bowl. Mash with a fork to mix and combine while still retaining some texture.
2. Pour melted coconut oil into mixture and blend in well.
3. Refrigirate mixture for 30 minutes, or until it solidifies.
4. Once the egg mixture is solid, remove from refrigerator and shape into 6 balls.
5. Wrap the balls in prosciutto slices.
6. Serve or refrigerate up to 4 days.

Salmon Mascarpone Balls

Prep time: 7 minutes

Cooking time: 0 minutes

Servings: 6

Nutrients per serving:

Carbohydrates – 1 g

Net Carbs – 0 g

Fat – 5 g

Protein – 3 g

Calories – 65

Ingredients:

- 3 oz smoked salmon, chopped
- 3 oz mascarpone
- ½ tsp maple flavor
- ½ tsp chives, chopped
- 3 Tbsp hemp hearts

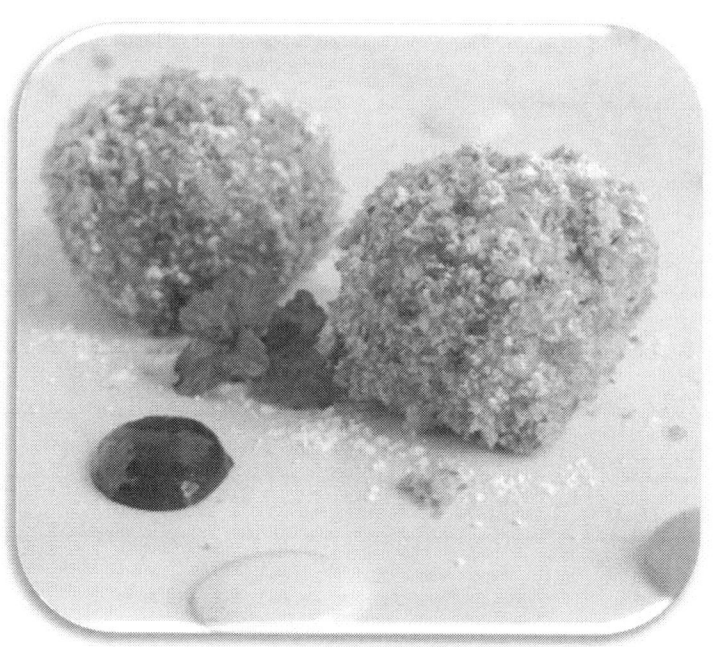

Instructions:

1. In a small food processor, combine salmon, mascarpone, maple flavor, and chives. Pulse a few times until blended together.
2. Form mixture into 6 balls.
3. Put hemp hearts on a medium plate and roll individual balls through to coat evenly.
4. Serve immediately or refrigerate up to 3 days.

Spicy Bacon and Avocado Balls

Prep time: 45 minutes

Cooking time: 8 minutes

Servings: 6

Nutrients per serving:

Carbohydrates – 3 g

Net Carbs – 1 g

Fat – 18 g

Protein – 3 g

Calories – 181

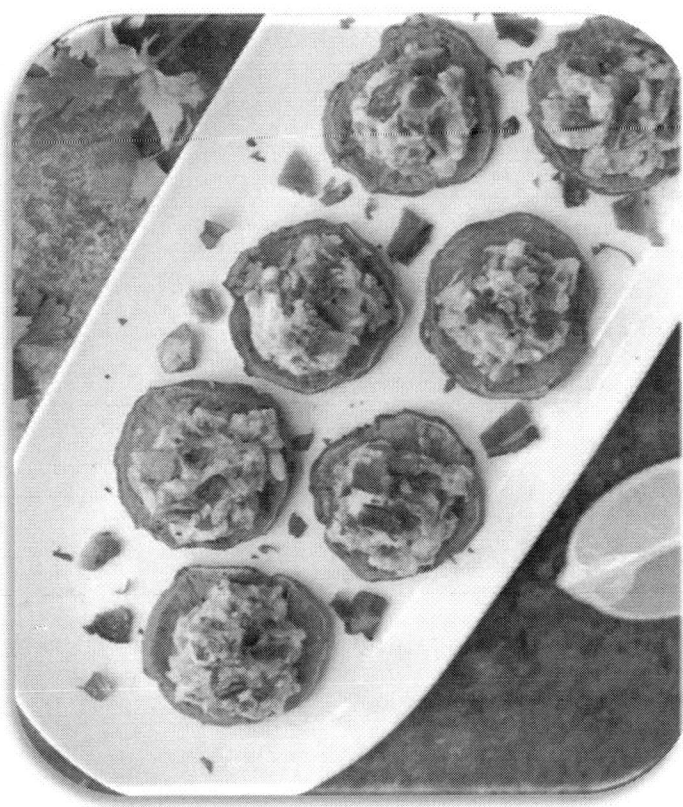

Ingredients:

- 4 slices bacon
- 1 medium avocado
- 2 Tbsp coconut oil
- 1 Tbsp bacon fat
- 1 Tbsp green onions, finely chopped
- 2 Tbsp cilantro, finely chopped
- 1 small jalapeño pepper, seeded, finely chopped
- ¼ tsp sea salt

Instructions:

1. Over medium heat, cook bacon until golden, about 4 minutes each side.
2. Drain bacon on a paper towel. Save bacon fat for later.
3. Once bacon is cool, chop 2 slices into crumbles.
4. Cut remaining 2 slices into 3 pieces each.
5. Smash avocado with a fork in a small bowl.
6. Add coconut oil and cooled bacon fat to avocado.
7. Add onion, cilantro, jalapeño, salt, and bacon crumbles. Blend well.
8. Refrigerate for 30 minutes.
9. Form mixture into 6 balls.
10. Place remaining 6 bacon pieces on a plate, then top each with an avocado ball.
11. Serve or refrigerate up to 3 days.

Salted Caramel and Brie Balls

Prep time: 5 minutes

Cooking time: 5 minutes

Servings: 6

Nutrients per serving:

Carbohydrates – 1 g

Net Carbs – 0 g

Fat – 12 g

Protein – 5 g

Calories – 130

Ingredients:

- 4 oz Brie, roughly chopped
- 2 oz salted macadamia nuts
- ½ tsp caramel flavor
- 1 Tbsp butter
- 1 large apple, chopped

Instructions:

1. In a food processor, mix all ingredients until a coarse mix forms, about 30 seconds.
2. Form mixture into 6 balls.

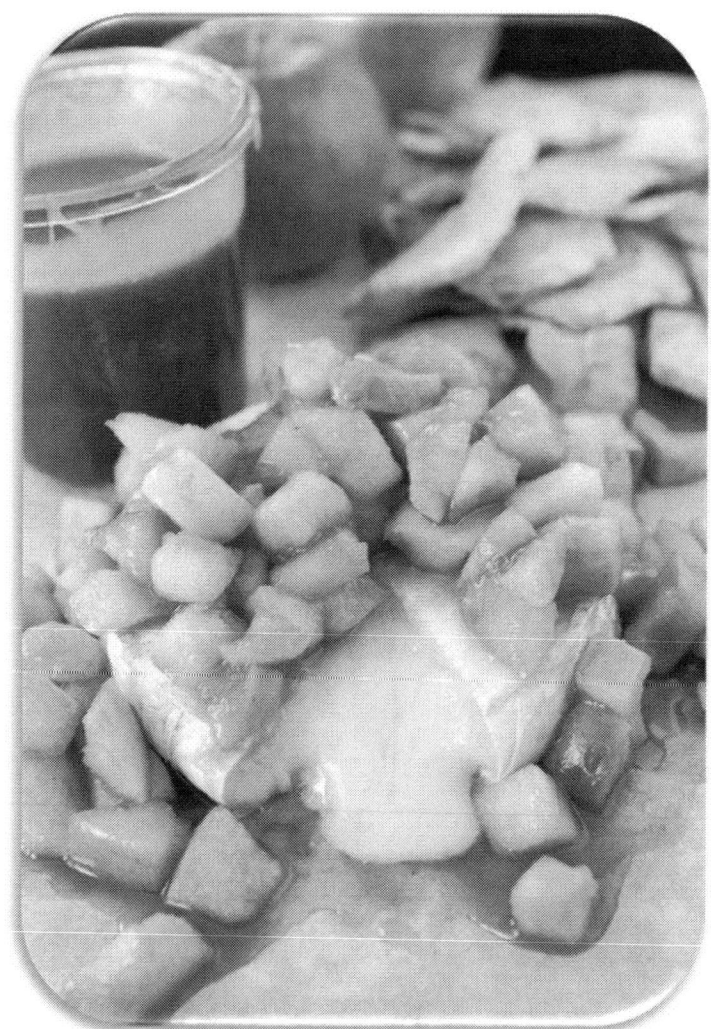

3. In a saucepan, melt the butter, then add the chopped apples. Cook until apples for about 5 minutes.
4. Spoon the apples over the brie balls. Serve or refrigerate up to 3 days.

Sunbutter Balls

Prep time: 20 minutes

Cooking time: 0 minutes

Servings: 12

Nutrients per serving:

Carbohydrates – 2 g

Net Carbs – 1 g

Fat – 13

Protein – 2 g

Calories – 124

Ingredients:

- 6 Tbsp mascarpone
- 3 Tbsp sunflower seed butter
- 6 Tbsp coconut oil, softened
- 3 Tbsp unsweetened shredded coconut flakes

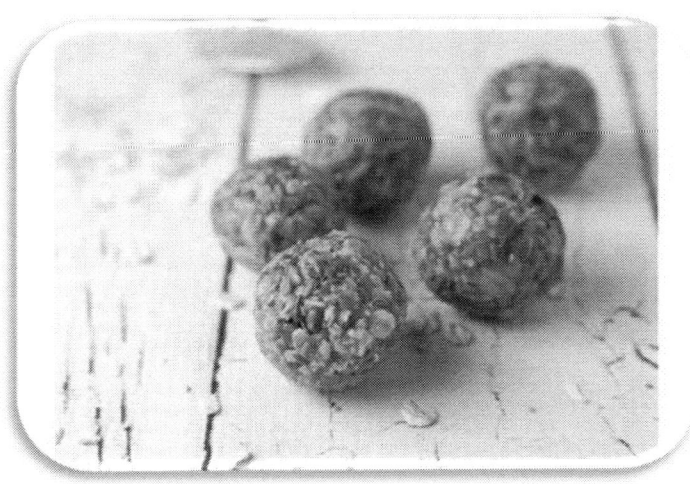

Instructions:

1. In a medium bowl, mix mascarpone, sunflower seed butter, and coconut oil until smooth paste forms.
2. Shape paste into walnut-sized balls.
3. Spread coconut flakes on a medium plate and roll individual balls through to coat evenly.

Baked Creamy Shrimps with Artichoke Hearts

Prep time: 5 minutes

Cooking time: 40 minutes

Servings: 16

Nutrients per serving:

Carbohydrates – 6.32 g

Net Carbs – 1.6 g

Fat – 11 g

Protein – 8 g

Calories – 150

Ingredients:

- 6 oz shrimp, precooked
- 2 Tbsp butter
- 1 can artichoke hearts, chopped
- 6 scallions
- ½ cup mayonnaise
- ½ cup sour cream
- 1 cup Cheddar cheese, shredded
- 1¼ cup Parmesan cheese, shredded
- 1 Tbsp garlic, minced
- 1 tsp red pepper flakes
- 1 tsp garlic powder

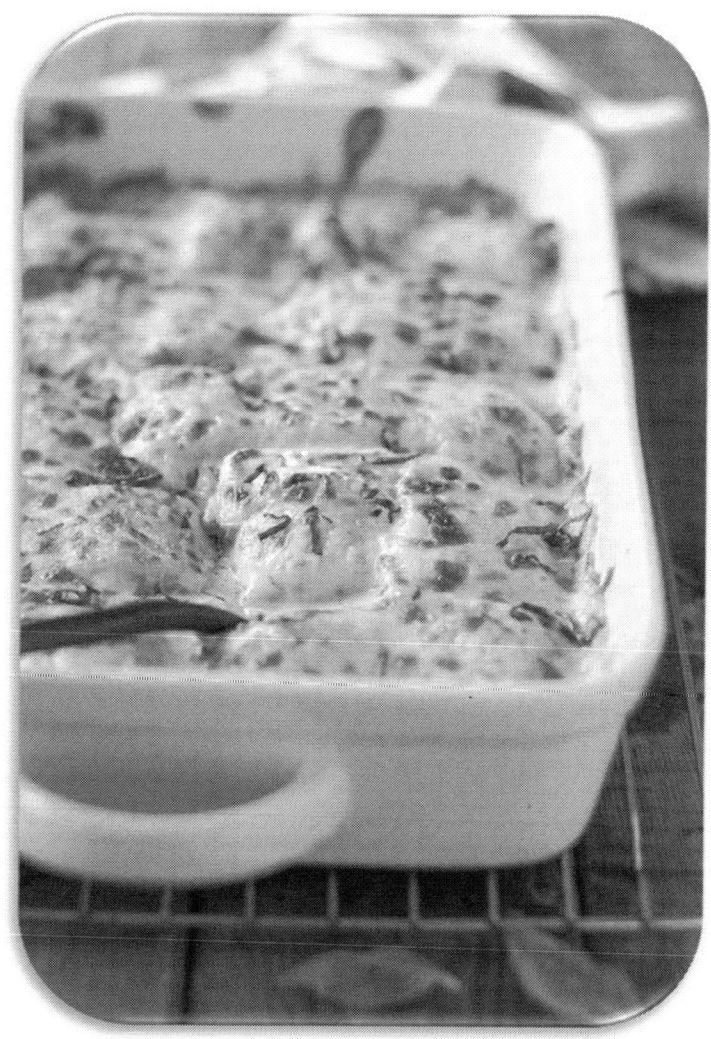

Instructions:

1. Preheat oven to 350°F.
2. In a frying pan, sauté shrimp over medium heat with butter and red pepper flakes for 5-10 minutes.
3. Chop the artichoke hearts.
4. In a bowl, combine all ingredient and mix well.
5. Pour the mixture in a baking dish and bake for 30 minutes. Serve hot.

Blue Cheese Turkey Dressed Eggs

Prep time: 1 hour 20 minutes

Cooking time: 12 minutes

Servings: 6

Nutrients per serving:

Carbohydrates – 3.9 g

Net Carbs – 0.6 g

Fat – 11.5 g

Protein – 14 g

Calories – 167

Ingredients:

- 6 hard-boiled eggs
- 2 green onions
- 6 oz smoked turkey breast, chopped
- ½ cup blue cheese, crumbled
- 2 Tbsp Blue cheese dressing
- ¼ cup mayonnaise
- 2 Tbsp hot mustard
- ½ rib celery

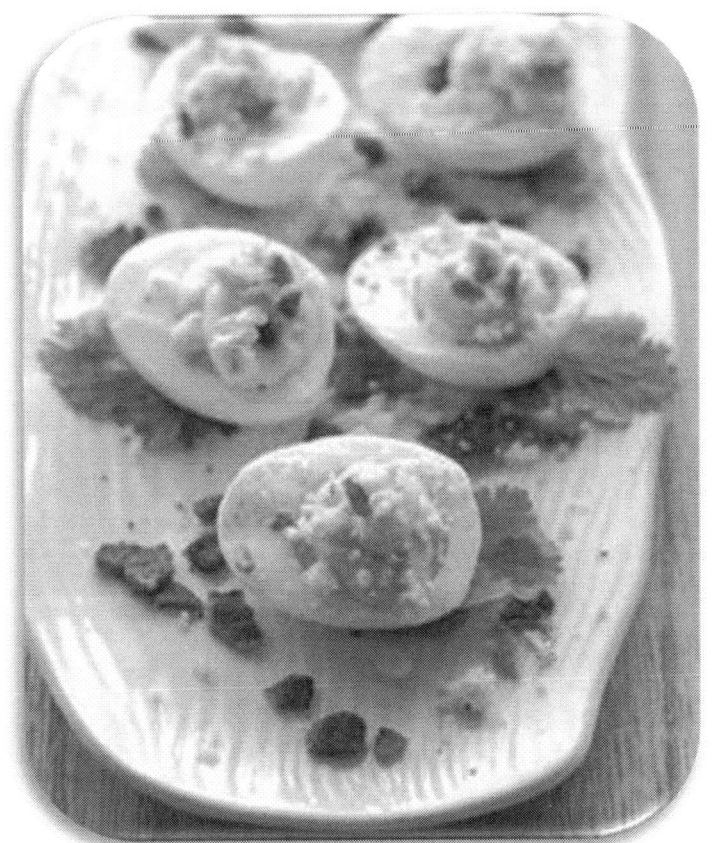

Instructions:

1. Chop smoked turkey breast and the celery.
2. Slice eggs in half lengthwise, scrape the yolks out into a bowl. Add the remaining ingredients except for the green onions.
3. Grate the green onions over the mixture. Mix all ingredients together.
4. With the teaspoon fill egg halves with the mixture.
5. Refrigerate for one hour. Serve.

Boiled Eggs and Pancetta Fat Bombs

Prep time: 20 minutes

Cooking time: 15 minutes

Servings: 4

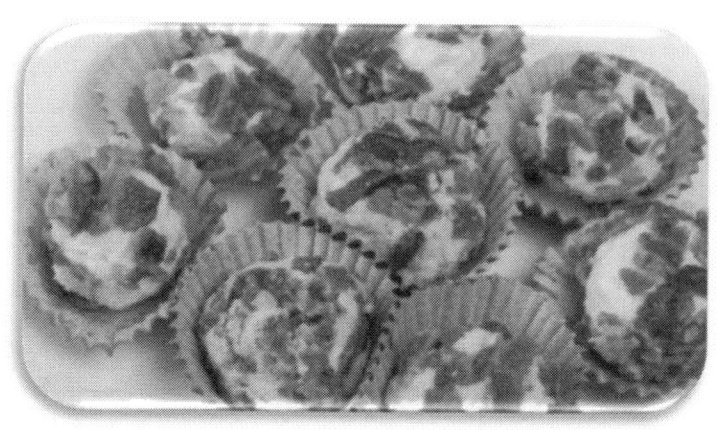

Nutrients per serving:

Carbohydrates – 2.2 g

Net Carbs – 0.5 g

Fat – 22 g

Protein – 7.5 g

Calories – 238

Ingredients:

- 4 large slices Pancetta
- 2 hard- boiled free-range eggs
- 1 cup ghee, softened
- 2 Tbsp mayonnaise
- Salt, freshly ground black pepper, to taste
- oconut oil for frying

Instructions:

1. Fry pancetta, 1-2 minutes per side. Remove from the fire and set aside.
2. In a deep bowl, combine ghee and eggs. Mash well with a fork. Add salt, pepper, and mayonnaise. Mix well. Refrigirate for one hour.
3. Make 4 equal balls.
4. Crumble the Pancetta into small pieces. Roll each ball in the Pancetta crumbles.
5. Refrigerate for 30 minutes more. Serve cold.

Olives and Sun-dried Tomatoes Fat Bombs

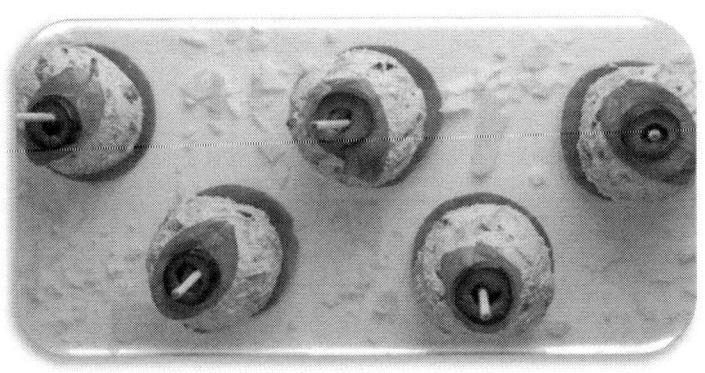

Prep time: 2 hours 20 minutes

Cooking time: 0 minutes

Servings: 4

Nutrients per serving:

Carbohydrates – 4 g

Net Carbs – 1 g

Fat – 14 g

Protein – 4.6 g

Calories – 157

Ingredients:

- 1 cup cream cheese
- 1 cup ghee
- 5 Tbsp Parmesan cheese, grated
- ¼ cup sun-dried tomatoes, chopped
- ¼ cup Kalamata olives, pitted
- 3 cloves garlic, crushed
- 3 Tbsp herbs mix (basil, parsley, thyme, oregano, parsnip, mint)
- Salt, freshly ground black pepper, to taste

Instructions:

1. In a bowl, mix the cream cheese and ghee. Set aside for 30-45 minutes to soften. Then mix to combine.
2. Add the chopped Kalamata olives and sun-dried tomatoes.
3. Add in herbs and crushed garlic; season with salt and pepper to taste. Mix well with and place the bowl in the fridge for at least 1 hour.
4. Take the cheese mixture out from the fridge and create 4 balls. Roll each ball in the Parmesan cheese.
5. Refrigerate for 30 minutes. Serve and enjoy.

Ham, Sausage, and Cashews Truffles

Prep time: 1 hour 15 minutes

Cooking time: 0 minutes

Servings: 12

Nutrients per serving:

Carbohydrates – 1.5 g

Net Carbs – 0.5 g

Fat – 11 g

Protein – 7 g

Calories – 125

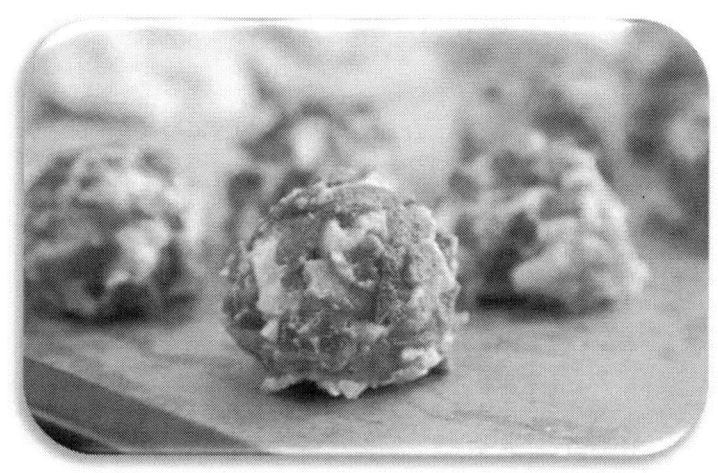

Ingredients:

- 8 slices smoked ham, finely chopped
- 8 oz sausages
- 6 oz cream cheese, softened
- 1 cup cashews, chopped
- 1 tsp Dijon mustard

Instructions:

1. In a food processor, blend sausages and cashews.
2. In a separate bowl, beat the cream cheese and mustard until soft.
3. Roll the sausage mixture into 12 small balls. Take each ball and form layer of cream cheese with your fingers.
4. Refrigerate for about 45-60 minutes.
5. Roll each ball in the finely chopped smoked ham and place on a serving dish. Serve.

Crab Cakes

Prep time: 40 minutes

Cooking time: 30 minutes

Servings: 4

Nutrition facts per serving:

Total carbs – 5 g

Protein – 19 g

Total fat – 10 g

Calories – 203

Ingredients:

- 1 lb crabmeat
- 1 egg
- 1 Tbsp Worcestershire sauce
- 1 Tbsp mayonnaise
- 1 Tbsp parsley
- Salt to taste

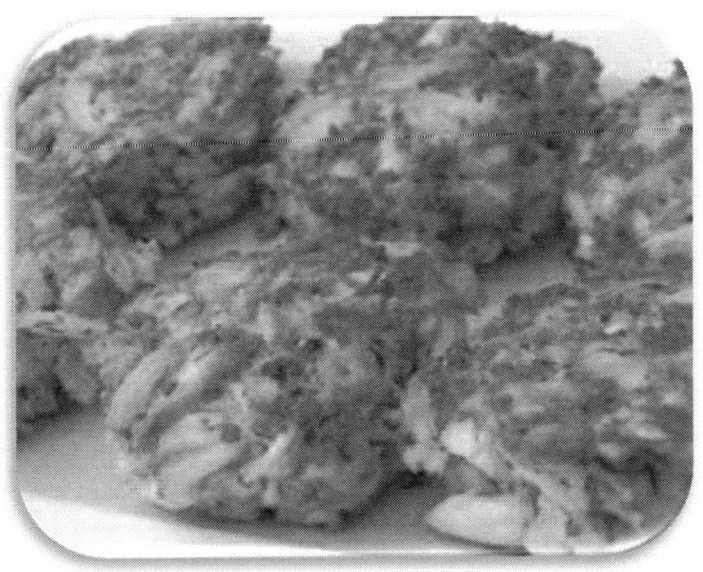

Instructions:

1. In a bowl mix together egg, Worcester- shire sauce, mayonnaise, parsley and season with salt.
2. Add in crabmeat, mix and form into cakes.
3. Place onto a baking sheet lined up with parchment paper.
4. Refrigerate for 30 minutes.
5. Bake for 30 minutes or until heated through at 375°F.

Sour Bacon Fat Bomb Dip

Prep time: 5 minutes

Cooking time: 30 minutes

Servings: 18

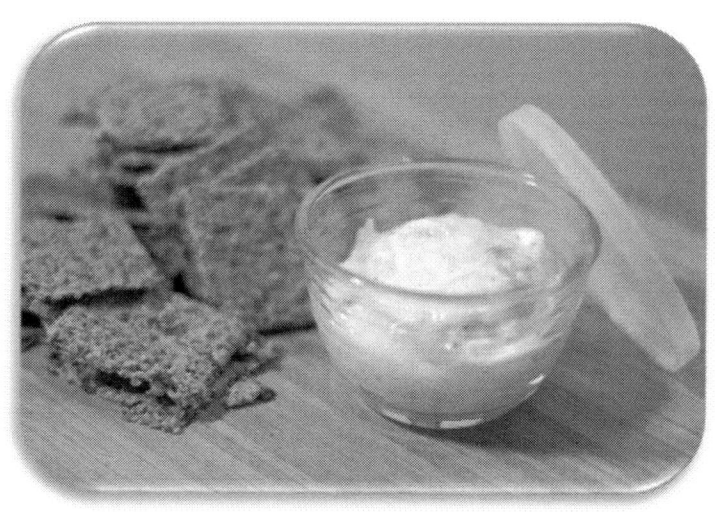

Nutrients per serving:

Carbohydrates – 1.7 g

Net Carbs – 1.4 g

Fat – 19 g

Protein – 5.5 g

Calories – 197

Ingredients:

- 6 slices bacon, cooked, crumbled
- 2 cups sour cream
- 1 cup cream cheese
- 1½ cups Cheddar cheese, shredded
- 1 cup sliced scallions

Instructions:

1. Preheat oven to 400°F.
2. In a deep bowl, combine all ingredients. Transfer mixture into a baking dish and bake until cheese is bubbling about 25-30 minutes.
3. Once ready, let cool and serve hot.

Turkey Bacon and Avocado Stuffed Eggs

Prep time: 1 hour 15 minutes

Cooking time: 12 minutes

Servings: 6

Nutrients per serving:

Carbohydrates – 4.4 g

Net Carbs – 0.5 g

Fat – 13 g

Protein – 9 g

Calories – 162

Ingredients:

- 6 hardb-boiled eggs
- 1 avocado
- 6 slices smoked turkey bacon
- 2 Tbsp mustard
- 1 Tbsp garlic, minced
- 1 Tbsp lime juice
- 1 Tbsp dried onion flakes
- Cayenne pepper, to taste
- 1 tsp garlic salt

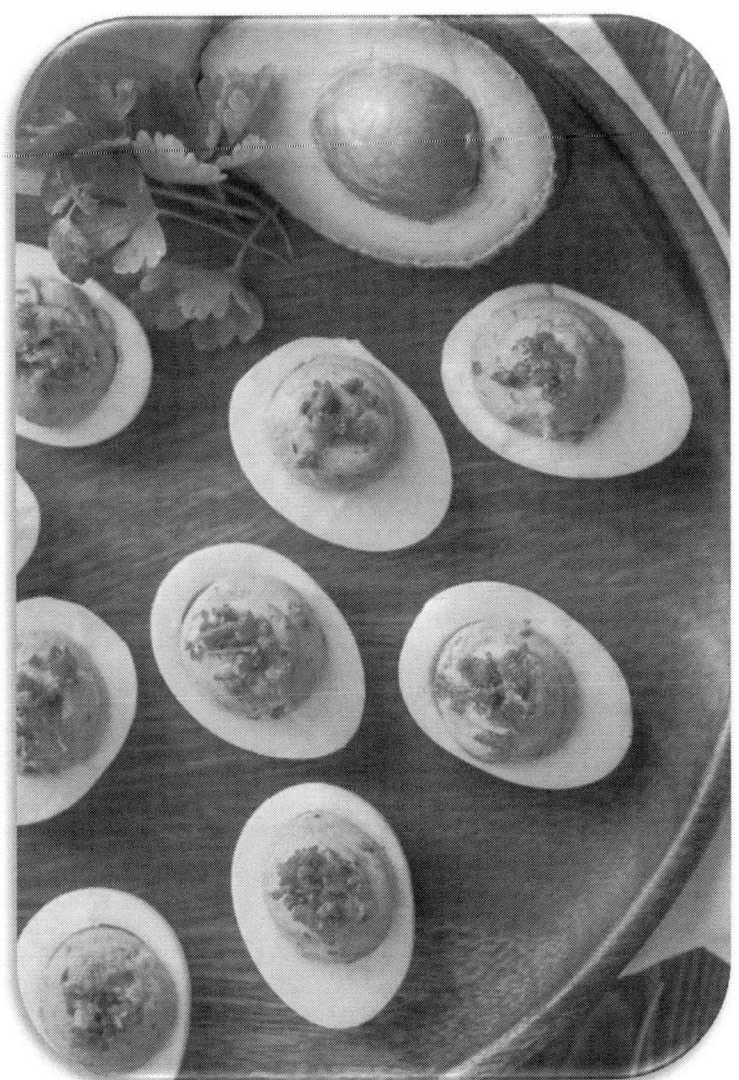

Instructions:

1. In a mixing bowl, mash the avocado.
2. Scrape the yolks out of the eggs and into the mixing bowl. Add in the bacon, mustard, cayenne pepper, lime juice, onion flakes, garlic and garlic salt. Mix well until smooth and creamy.
3. Fill each egg half with the avocado mixture. Refrigerate stuffed eggs for 1 hour. Serve.

Viva Mexico Angels Eggs

Prep time: 1 hour 20 minutes

Cooking time: 12 minutes

Servings: 6

Nutrients per serving:

Carbohydrates – 4.5 g

Net Carbs – 0.2 g

Fat – 13.5 g

Protein – 7 g

Calories – 163

Ingredients:

- ¼ cup cream cheese, softened
- 6 slices Pancetta
- 6 large hard-boiled eggs
- 6 Tbsp mayonnaise
- 16 sliced pickled Guajillo chili peppers
- ¼ tsp smoked paprika

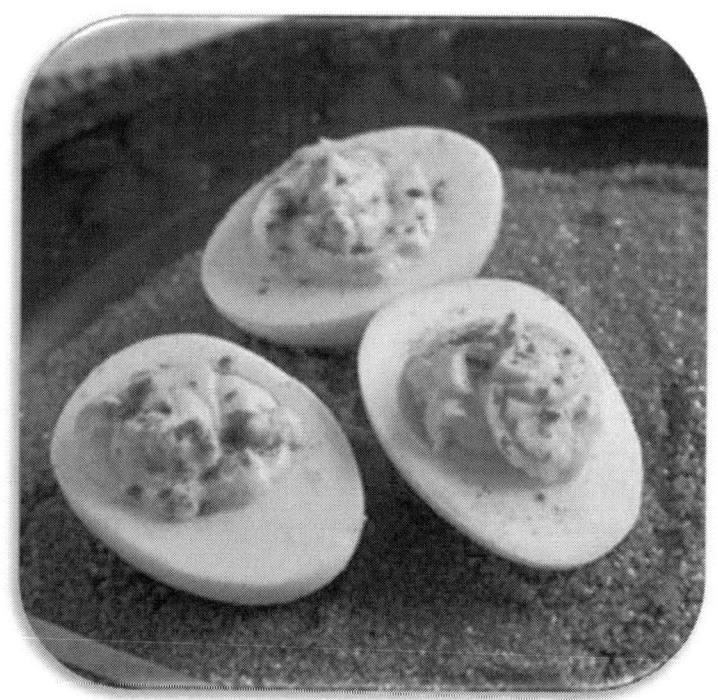

Instructions:

1. Chop 4 of the Guajillo chilis and set aside.
2. Remove yolks from hard-boiled eggs and mash them in a medium bowl.
3. Add pancetta, mayonnaise, cream cheese, and chopped Guajillo chili to the bowl. Mix until all ingredients are well incorporated.
4. Fill the egg halves with the mixter and top each egg with a Guajillo chili slice.
5. Sprinkle with paprika and refrigerate for 1 hour. Serve.

Hot Hot Fat Bombs

Prep time: 20 minutes

Cooking time: 5 minutes

Servings: 6

Nutrients per serving:

Carbohydrates – 1.3 g

Net Carbs – 0.6 g

Fat – 16 g

Protein – 4 g

Calories – 165

Ingredients:

- ½ cup Cream cheese
- 4 slices Pepperoni Sausages
- 3 slices smoked bacon
- 1 medium chili pepper
- ½ tsp dried basil
- ¼ tsp onion powder
- ¼ tsp garlic powder
- Salt, pepper, to taste

Instructions:

1. In a frying pan, brown bacon and Peperoni sausages until crisp.
2. Remove bacon and Pepperoni from the pan on a paper lined plate to cool. Keep the remaining grease for later use.
3. Dice chili pepper into small pieces.

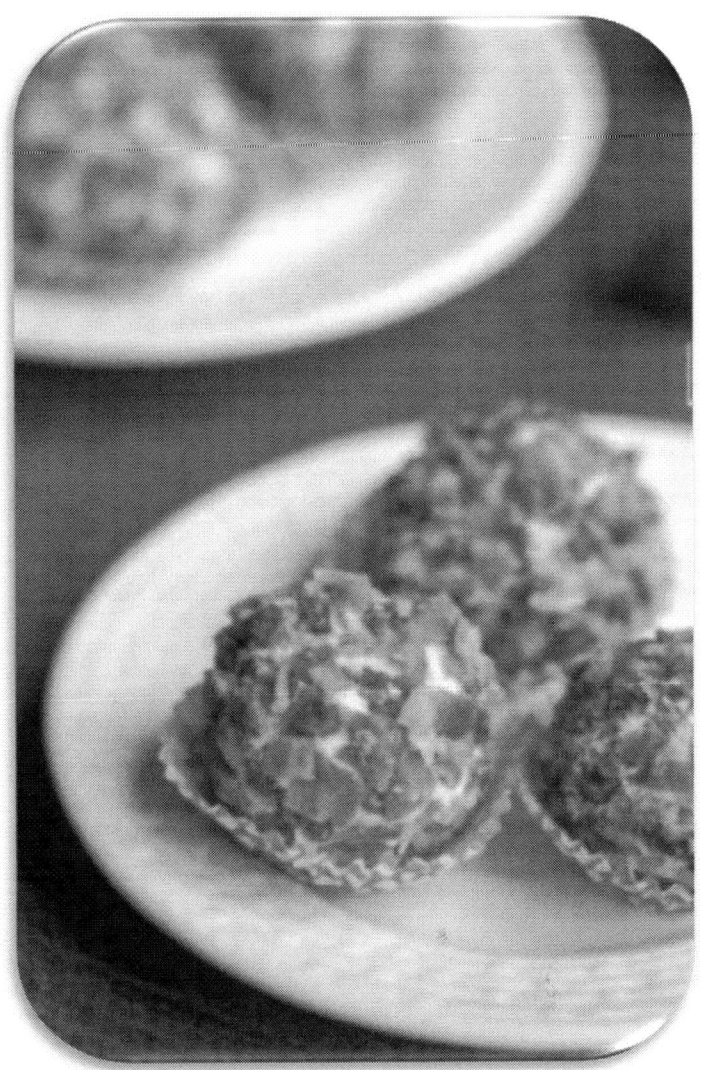

4. Combine cream cheese, chilli pepper, and spices. Add the bacon fat in and mix together until a solid mixture is formed. Season with salt and pepper to taste.
5. Crumble bacon and Pepperone slices and set on a plate. Roll cream cheese mixture into 6 balls, then roll the ball into the bacon or Pepperone.

Wrapped Bacon Rolls

Prep time: 10 minutes

Cooking time: 0 minutes

Servings: 12

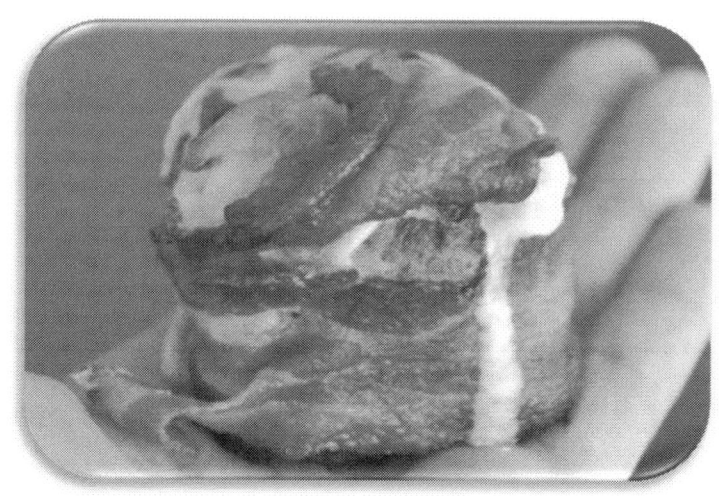

Nutrients per serving:

Carbohydrates – 2.7 g

Net Carbs – 0.7 g

Fat – 17.7 g

Protein – 1.78 g

Calories – 174

Ingredients:

- 4 bacon slices
- 6 toasted pecan halves, chopped
- ½ cup unsalted butter
- ½ cup mayonnaise
- Granulated garlic, to taste

Instructions:

1. Divide each bacon slice into 3 equal parts.
2. Spread each bacon slice with unsalted butter. Press pecan pieces into butter.
3. Top with each with mayonnaise, sprinkle with granulated garlic and wrap in rolls. Serve.

Pancetta Wrapped Provolone Sticks

Prep time: 10 minutes

Cooking time: 3 minutes

Servings: 10

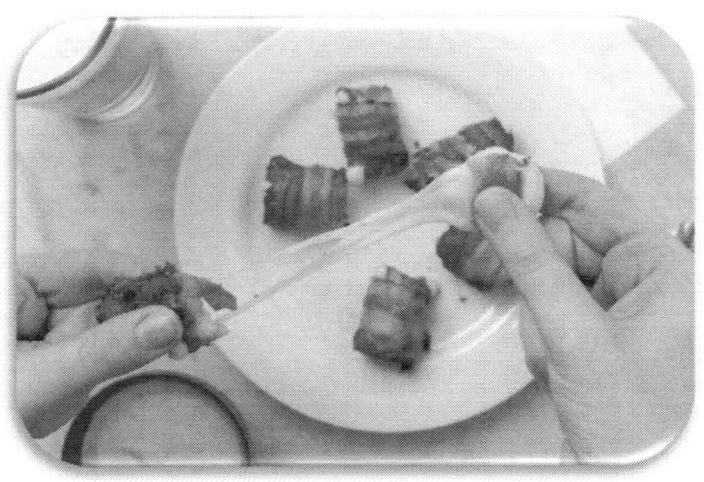

Nutrients per serving:

Carbohydrates – 0.42 g

Net Carbs – 0.08 g

Fat – 22 g

Protein – 5.6 g

Calories – 216

Ingredients:

- 4 slices Pancetta bacon
- 2 Frigo string Provolone cheese (or Mozzarela, Kasseri, Emmenthal)
- ½ cup coconut oil for frying

Instructions:

1. Preheat coconut oil to 350°F in a deep fryer.
2. Wrap Provolone around Pancetta and secure with a toothpick.
3. Drop the bacon wrapped cheese in the hot oil and cook about 2-3 minutes, depending on the thickness of your bacon.
4. Remove to a paper towel to cool for a few minutes. Remove the toothpick and serve.

Savory Coco Bacon Fat Bombs

Prep time: 40 minutes

Cooking time: 0 minutes

Servings: 24

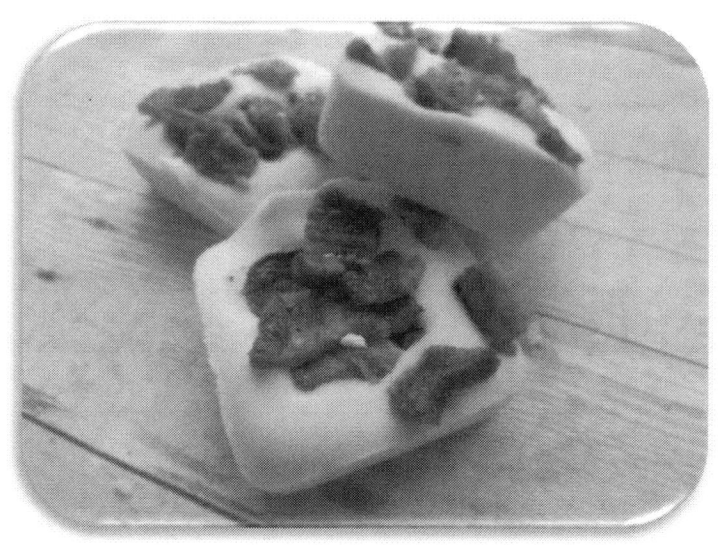

Nutrients per serving:

Carbohydrates – 0.5 g

Net Carbs – 0.3 g

Fat – 15.9 g

Protein – 0 g

Calories – 261

Ingredients:

- 8 strips cooked crispy bacon, crumbled, divided
- 1 cup cream cheese, softened
- ½ cup butter
- 4 tsp bacon fat
- 4 Tbsp coconut oil
- ¼ cup Splenda

Instructions:

1. In a microwave-safe dish, combine all ingredients and melt slowly in the microwave until smooth. Set aside 1 bacon strip.
2. Pour into a dish or pan and freeze until firm, about 30 minutes.
3. Before serving, remove from freezer, sprinkle with crumbled bacon, slice and serve.

Greek-Style Fat Bomb Balls

Prep time: 20 minutes

Cooking time: 0 minutes

Servings: 5

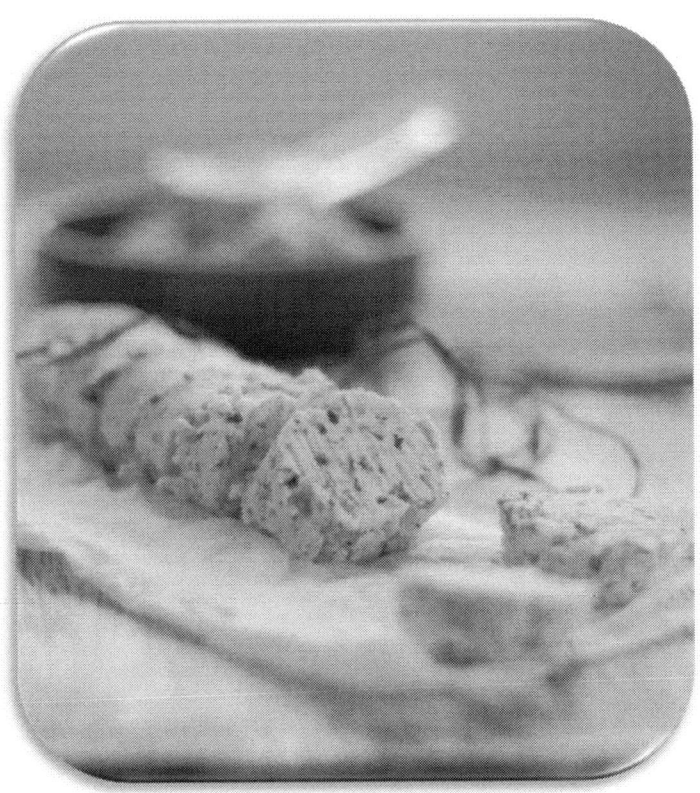

Nutrients per serving:

Carbohydrates – 2.8 g

Net Carbs – 0.8 g

Fat – 19.8 g

Protein – 3.67 g

Calories – 200

Ingredients:

- 1 cup cream cheese, softened
- 1 cup butter, softened
- 2-3 Tbsp freshly chopped herbs (any combination of basil, thyme, oregano and/or parsley works great) or 2 tsp of dried herbs
- 4 sun-dried tomatoes, drained
- 4 Kalamata olives, pitted, chopped
- 2 cloves garlic, crushed
- Black pepper, to taste
- 1 tsp sea salt
- 5 Tbsp Parmesan cheese, finely grated

Instructions:

1. Mash the butter and cream cheese together with a fork and mix until well combined. Mix in the sun-dried tomatoes and Kalamata olives.

2. Stir in the herbs, garlic, salt, and pepper. Mix and refrigirate for 20-30 minutes.

3. Make 5 balls out from the mixture. A spoon or an ice-cream scooper works well.

4. Place the grated Parmesan cheese in a shallow dish. Roll each ball in the cheese and place on a plate. Serve or store in the fridge in an airtight container for up to a week.

Scrambled Eggs Muffins

Prep time: 45 minutes

Cooking time: 0 minutes

Servings: 8

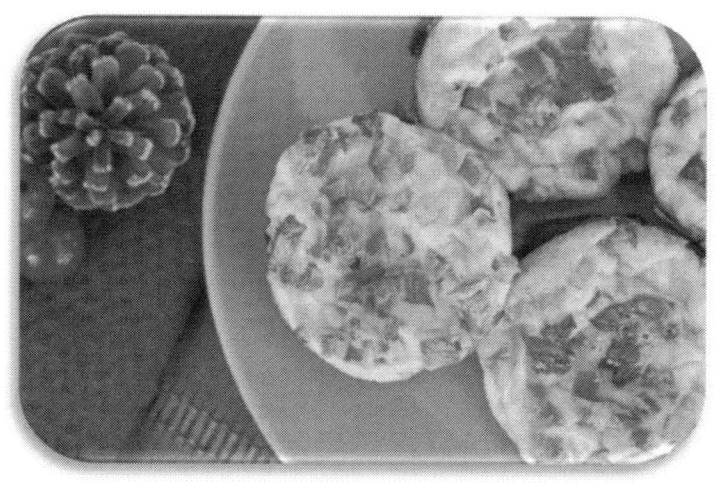

Nutrients per serving:

Carbohydrates – 0.54 g

Net Carbs – 0.3 g

Fat – 16.9 g

Protein – 7.9 g

Calories – 186

Ingredients:

- 3 strips bacon, cooked, crumbled
- 6 six eggs
- 2 Tbsp coconut oil or butter
- 1 Tbsp butter
- ¼ cup softened cream cheese
- ¼ cup Gouda cheese, shredded

Instructions:

1. In a small bowl, melt the butter and set aside. In a separate bowl, beat the eggs. Add in spices. Melt some butter in a non stick skillet on medium heat and scramble the eggs.
2. Put cooked eggs into another large bowl. Mix in cheeses. Add bacon and stir. Add the melted butter and coconut oil.
3. Pour the batter in mini muffin liners. Place on cookie sheet with or without wax paper, and freeze for about 30 minutes. Serve.

Simple Parmesan Crisps

Prep time: 15 minutes

Cooking time: 15 minutes

Servings: 4

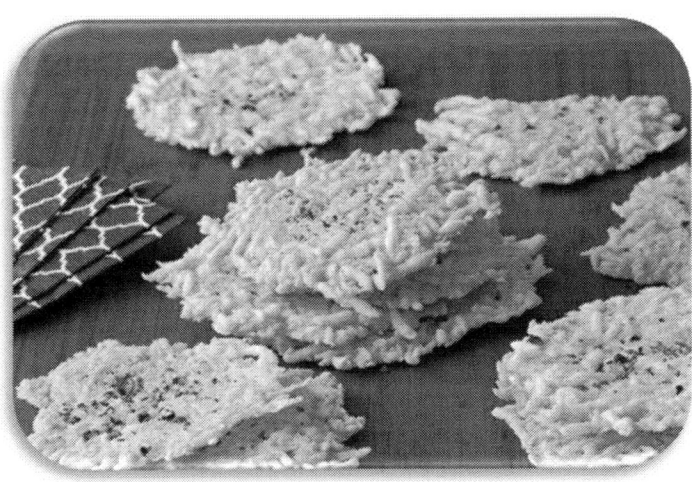

Nutrients per serving:

Carbohydrates – 6.45 g

Net Carbs – 0.35 g

Fat – 7.47 g

Protein – 10.4 g

Calories – 135.5

Ingredients:

- 1 cup parmesan cheese
- 4 Tbsp coconut flour
- 1-2 tsp rosemary, oregano, or any herbs of choice, dried or fresh

Instructions:

1. Preheat the oven to 350°F. In a small bowl, combine all ingredients.
2. Scoop one teaspoon at a time of the cheese mixture onto a baking tray lined with parchment paper, leaving a small gap between each. Place in the oven and cook for 10-15 minutes, or until golden brown. Be careful not to burn.
3. Remove from the oven and let cool for 15 minutes. Serve

Smoked Sardine Paté

Prep time: 10 minutes

Cooking time: 5 minutes

Servings: 8

Nutrition facts per serving:

Total carbs – 2 g

Protein – 9.4 g

Total fat – 7.3 g

Calories –106

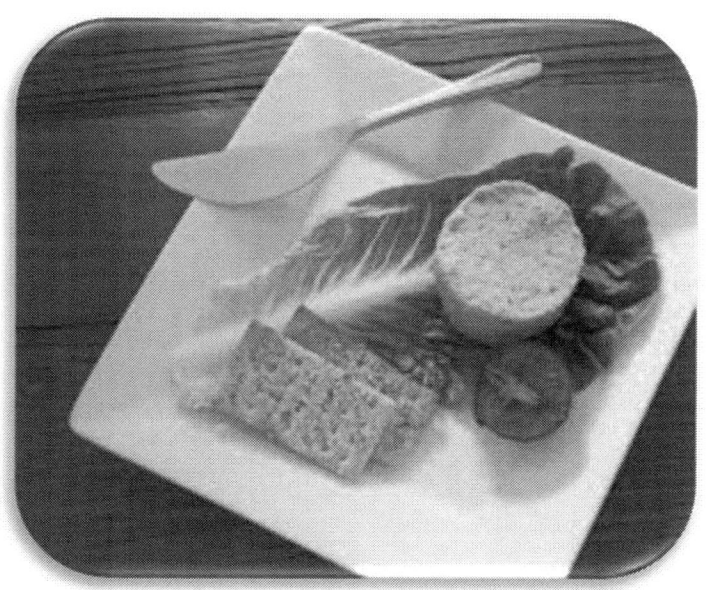

Ingredients:

- 2 cans (6.7 oz) smoked sardines
- 1 cup cottage cheese
- 7 oz Greek yogurt
- 2 Tbsp lemon juice

Instructions:

1. Add the sardines to a food processor. Add in cottage cheese, Greek yogurt and lemon juice.
2. Blend until smooth.
3. Transfer to a bowl and keep refrigerated.
4. Serve on spinach or lettuce leaves.

Tuna & Olive Endive Cups

Prep time: 5 minutes

Cooking time: 0 minutes

Servings: 4

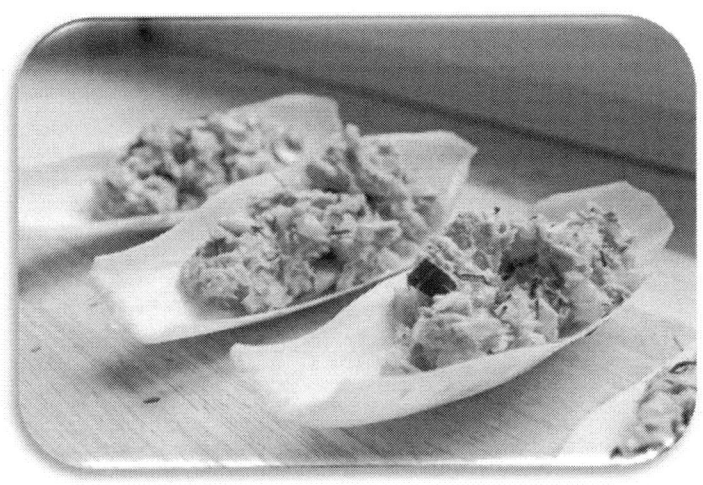

Nutrients per serving:

Carbohydrates – 1 g

Net Carbs –0 g

Fat – 2 g

Protein – 2 g

Calories – 29

Ingredients:

- 1 oz canned tuna in olive oil, drained
- 6 large kalamata olives, pitted
- ½ Tbsp chopped green onion
- 1 tsp extra-virgin olive oil
- 4 Belgian endive leaves, washed and dried

Instructions:

1. In a food processor, combine all ingredients.
2. Scoop 1 Tbsp tuna mix onto each endive leaf.
3. Serve.

Creamy Tuna Endive Cups

Prep time: 5 minutes

Cooking time: 0 minutes

Servings: 4

Nutrients per serving:

Carbohydrates – 2 g

Net Carbs –1 g

Fat – 3 g

Protein – 3 g

Calories – 46

Ingredients:

- 1 oz canned tuna in olive oil, drained
- 1 oz cream cheese
- 4 Belgian endive leaves, washed and dried
- 2 Tbsp hemp hearts

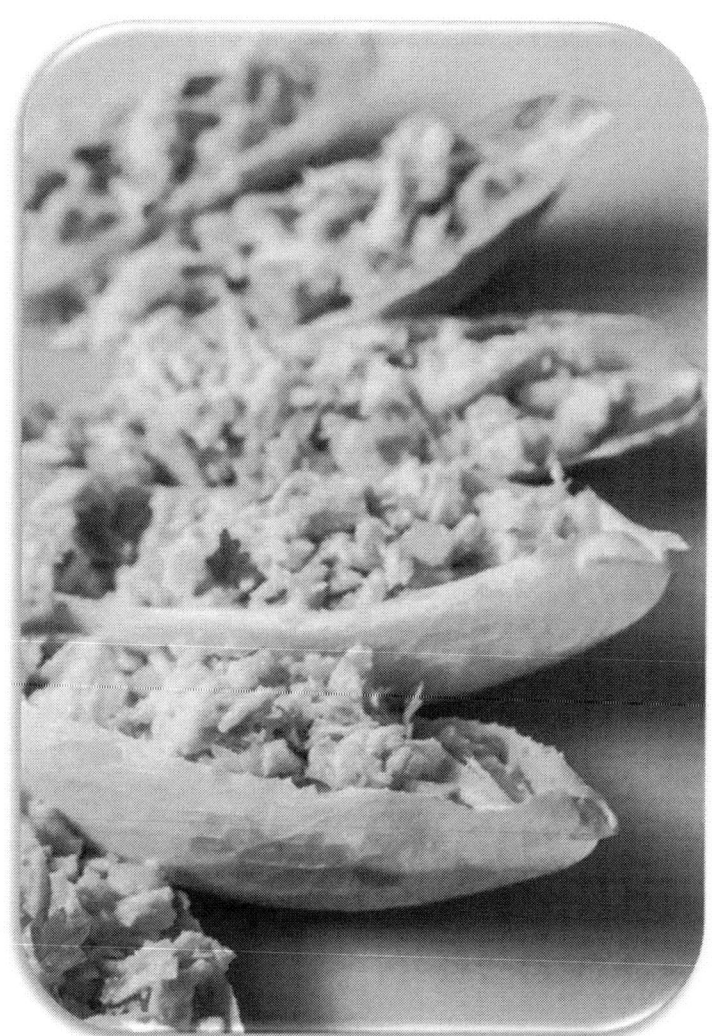

Instructions:

1. In a small food processor, mix tuna and cream cheese until well blended.
2. Scoop 1 Tbsp tuna cream onto each endive cup.
3. Sprinkle ½ Tbsp hemp hearts over each endive cup. Serve immediately.

Nutty Bacon Baskets

Prep time: 15 minutes

Cooking time: 20 minutes

Servings: 6

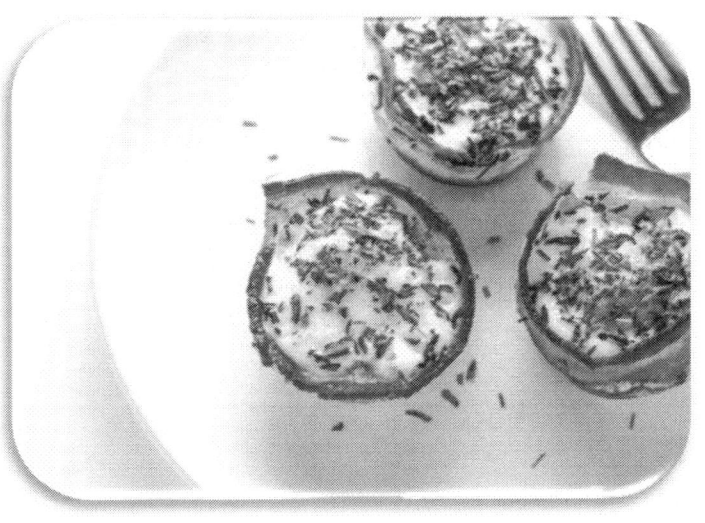

Nutrients per serving:

Carbohydrates – 3 g

Net Carbs – 1.54 g

Fat – 44 g

Protein – 9 g

Calories – 437

Ingredients:

- 12 slices bacon, 6 cut in half
- 4 slices cooked bacon, chopped into bits
- 1 Tbsp butter
- ½ cup pecans
- ½ cup macadamia nuts
- ¼ tsp granulated garlic
- 1/8 tsp freshly ground black pepper

Instructions:

1. Preheat oven to 400°F.
2. In a standard-sized muffin tin, place half-strips bacon in an X shape in the bottom of 6 cups. Line those same cups with 1 full slice bacon along with the inside of the cup vertically.
3. Place a cookie sheet underneath muffin tin and bake cups 15 minutes until slightly browned and crisp.
4. While cups are baking, melt butter over medium-low heat in a medium skillet. Add nuts, garlic, and pepper and cook 4-5 minutes. Remove from heat.
5. Once cooled, coarsely chop nut mixture and combine with bacon bits.
6. Divide nut mixture between cups and serve.

Olive Dynamite Prosciutto Cup

Prep time: 20 minutes

Cooking time: 12 minutes

Servings: 1

Nutrients per serving:

Carbohydrates – 8 g

Net Carbs – 4 g

Fat – 16 g

Protein – 8 g

Calories – 209

Ingredients:

- 1 slice prosciutto
- 1 medium egg yolk
- 1 Tbsp olive oil mayonnaise
- 4 large kalamata olives, pitted and chopped
- ¼ tsp Herbes de Provence

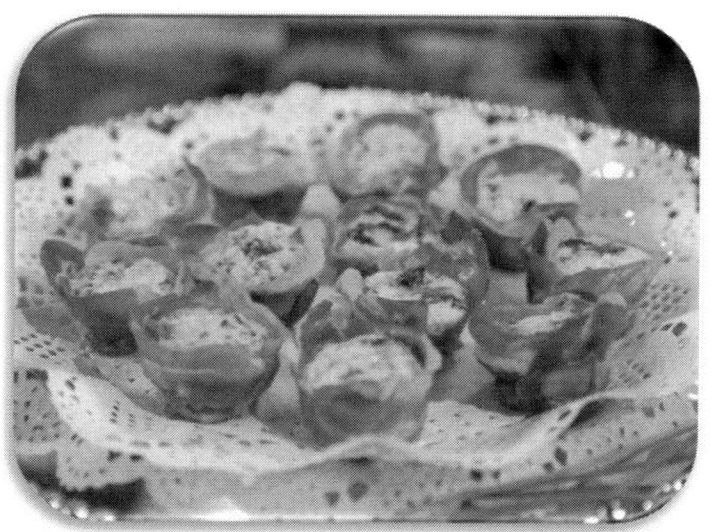

Instructions:

1. Preheat oven to 350°F.
2. Fold prosciutto slice in half, so it becomes almost square.
3. Place it in a muffin tin hole to line it completely.
4. Place egg yolk into prosciutto cup.
5. Gently place mayonnaise and olives on top of the egg. Sprinkle with Herbes de Provence.
6. Bake about 12 minutes, until egg yolk is still runny but warm.
7. Set aside for 15 minutes before removing from muffin pan.

Baked Brie and Pecan Prosciutto Cup

Prep time: 20 minutes

Cooking time: 12 minutes

Servings: 1

Nutrients per serving:

Carbohydrates – 2 g

Net Carbs – 1 g

Fat – 15 g

Protein – 12 g

Calories – 182

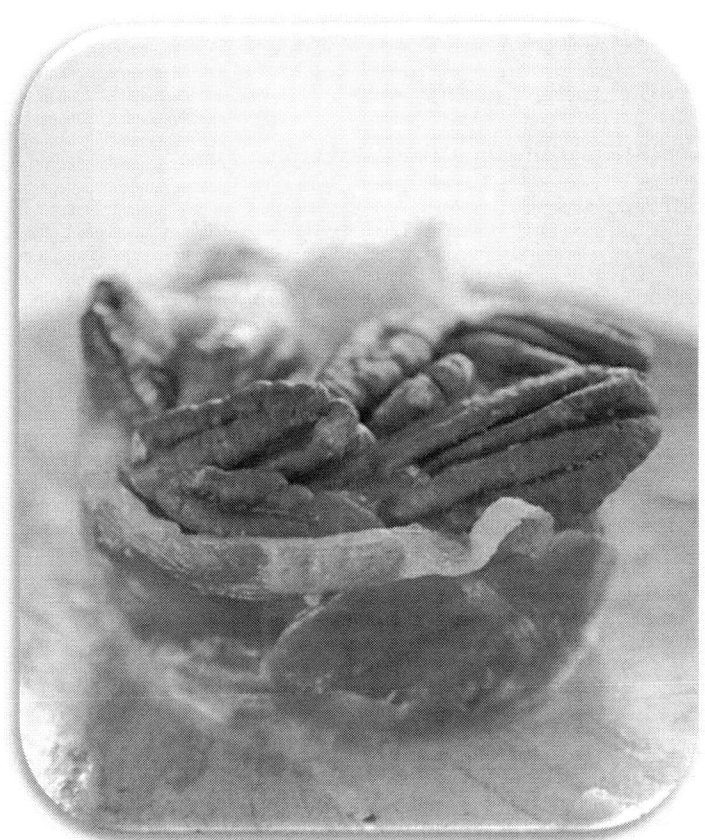

Ingredients:

- 1 slice prosciutto
- 1 oz Brie, diced with white skin on
- 6 pecan halves
- 1/8 tsp freshly ground black pepper

Instructions:

1. Preheat oven to 350°F.
2. Fold prosciutto slice in half, so it becomes almost square.
3. Place it in muffin tin hole to line it completely.
4. Place Brie in the prosciutto-lined cup.
5. Stick pecan halves in amongst Brie.
6. Bake about 12 minutes, until Brie is melted and prosciutto is cooked.
7. Let cool 10 minutes before removing from muffin pan.

Cheesy Muffin Prosciutto Cup

Prep time: 20 minutes

Cooking time: 12 minutes

Servings: 1

Nutrients per serving:

Carbohydrates – 2 g

Net Carbs – 1 g

Fat – 15 g

Protein – 18 g

Calories – 218

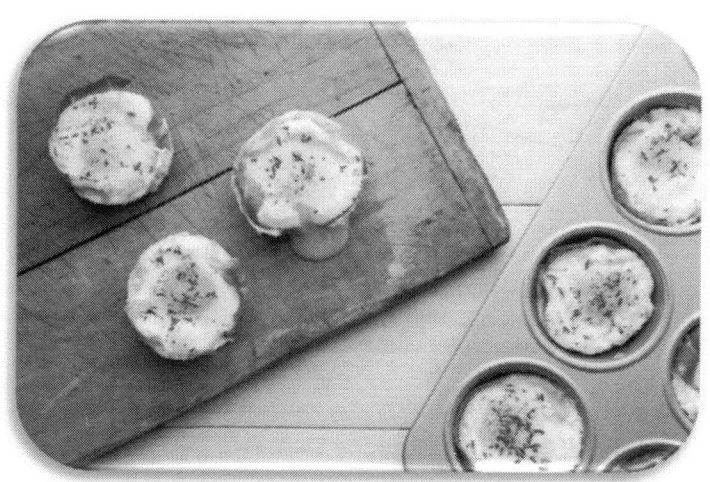

Ingredients:

- 1 slice prosciutto
- 1 medium egg yolk
- ½ oz diced Brie
- 1/3 oz diced mozzarella
- ½ oz grated Parmesan

Instructions:

1. Preheat oven to 350°F.
2. Fold prosciutto slice in half, so it becomes almost square.
3. Place it in muffin tin hole to line it completely.
4. Place egg yolk into prosciutto cup.
5. Add cheeses on top of egg yolk without breaking it.
6. Bake about 12 minutes, until yolk is cooked and warm but still runny.
7. Set aside for 15 minutes before removing from muffin pan.

Quattro Formaggi Rollups

Prep time: 5 minutes

Cooking time: 5 minutes

Servings: 2

Nutrients per serving:

Carbohydrates –1 g

Net Carbs –1 g

Fat – 13 g

Protein – 9 g

Calories – 152

Ingredients:

- 1 large egg
- 1 Tbsp Parmesan, grated
- 1 Tbsp blue cheese, crumbled
- 1 tsp butter
- 1 Tbsp mascarpone
- 1 oz Brie, thinly sliced

Instructions:

1. In a small bowl, whisk egg, Parmesan, and blue cheese until foamy.
2. Heat a small nonstick skillet over high heat and melt butter.
3. Pour in egg mixture, spreading evenly, so it forms a thin, even layer.

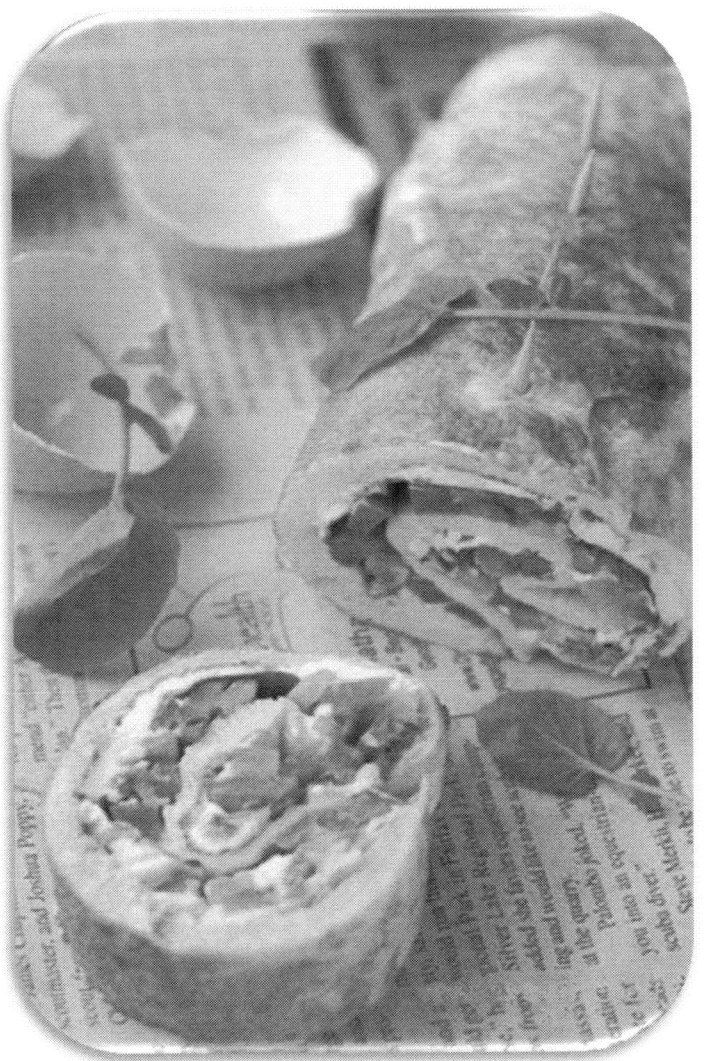

4. Once the first side is cooked, about 1 minute, flip frittata.
5. Spread mascarpone on top of the frittata, then place Brie slices in the middle and cover with a lid.
6. Cook until golden on bottom, about 2 more minutes.
7. Remove frittata to a plate.
8. Roll frittata into a tight roll, cut into 2 pieces and serve immediately while hot.

Mascarpone Balls

Prep time: 20 minutes

Cooking time: 0 minutes

Servings: 12

Nutrients per serving:

Carbohydrates –2 g

Net Carbs –1 g

Fat –13

Protein – 2 g

Calories – 124

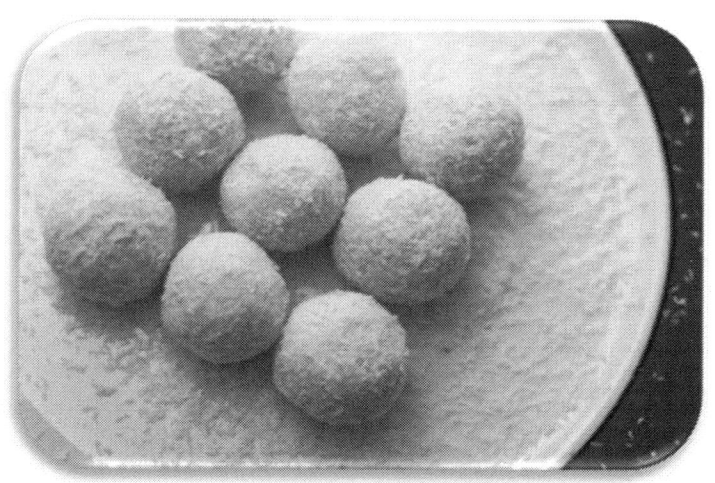

Ingredients:

- 6 Tbsp mascarpone
- 3 Tbsp sunflower seed butter
- 6 Tbsp coconut oil, softened
- 3 Tbsp unsweetened shredded coconut flakes

Instructions:

1. In a medium bowl, mix mascarpone, sunflower seed butter, and coconut oil until smooth paste forms.
2. Shape paste into 12 walnut-sized balls.
3. Spread coconut flakes on a medium plate and roll individual balls through to coat evenly.

Salami & Olive Rollups

Prep time: 5 minutes

Cooking time: 0 minutes

Servings: 3

Nutrients per serving:

Carbohydrates – 6 g

Net Carbs – 2.4 g

Fat – 20 g

Protein – 8 g

Calories – 233

Ingredients:

- 12 large kalamata olives, pitted
- 3 oz cream cheese
- 3 (1-oz) slices Italian salami

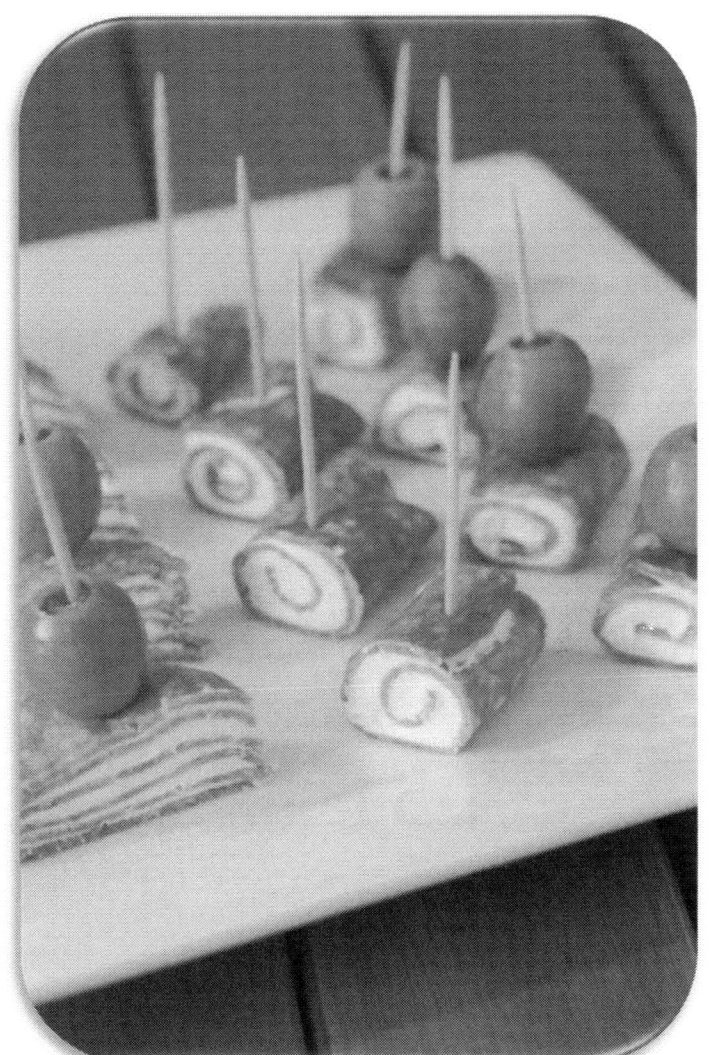

Instructions:

1. In a small food processor, mix olives and cream cheese until they form a coarse mixture, about 10 seconds.
2. Form cheese mixture into 3 balls.
3. Place each ball on a slice of salami, then roll salami around it and secure with a toothpick.
4. Serve or refrigerate up to 3 days.

Smoked Salmon & Avocado Rollups

Prep time: 5 minutes

Cooking time: 0 minutes

Servings: 3

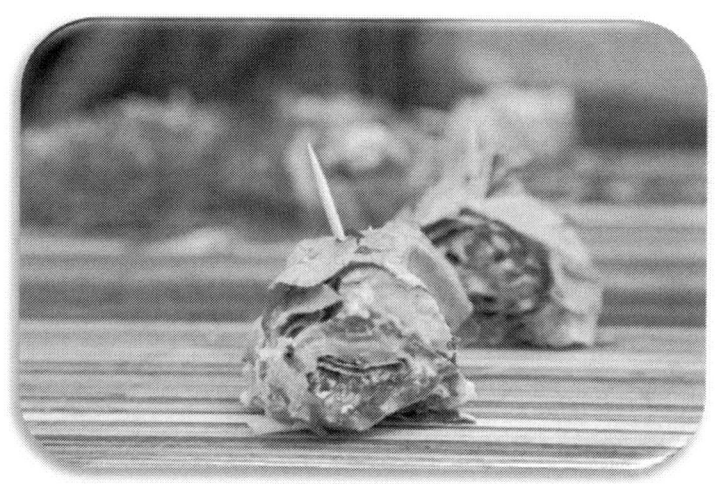

Nutrients per serving:

Carbohydrates – 2 g

Net Carbs – 0 g

Fat – 5 g

Protein – 6 g

Calories – 78

Ingredients:

- 3 oz avocado flesh
- 1 tsp fresh lemon juice
- 1/8 tsp sea salt
- 3 slices smoked salmon (lox), about 1 oz each

Instructions:

1. In a bowl, combine avocado, lemon juice, and salt.
2. Spread avocado mixture evenly on top of each salmon slice.
3. Roll slices into individual rolls and secure with a toothpick.
4. Serve immediately.

Mediterranean Rollups

Prep time: 7 minutes

Cooking time: 3 minutes

Servings: 2

Nutrients per serving:

Carbohydrates – 14 g

Net Carbs – 4 g

Fat – 10 g

Protein –5 g

Calories – 153

Ingredients:

- 1 large egg
- 1 Tbsp extra-virgin olive oil
- 1/8 tsp sea salt
- 6 large kalamata olives, pitted
- 1 oz sun-dried tomatoes in oil
- 1/8 tsp red chili flakes
- 1/8 tsp parsley flakes

Instructions:

1. In a small bowl, combine egg, olive oil, and salt, and whisk until foamy.
2. Heat a small nonstick skillet over high heat and pour in egg mixture, spreading evenly, so it forms a thin, even layer.

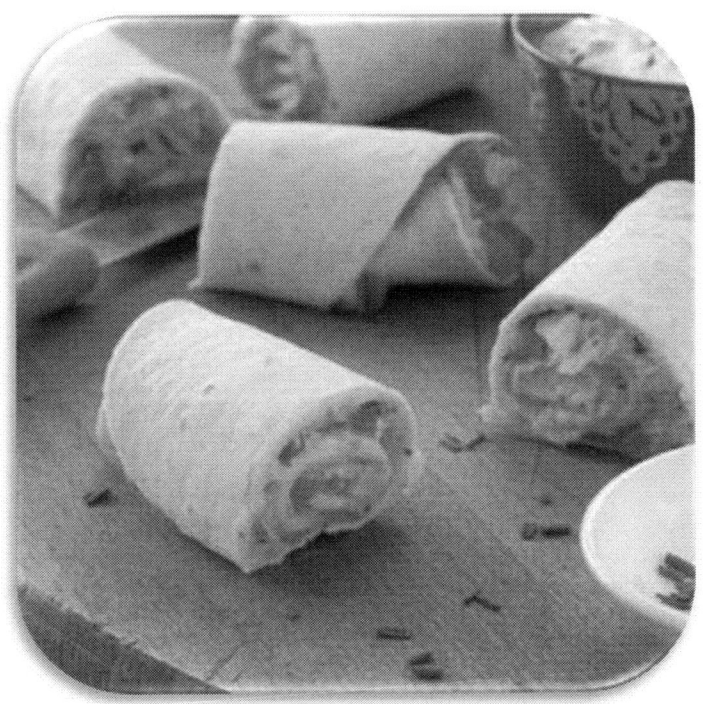

3. Once the first side is cooked, about 1 minute, flip frittata and cook until golden on bottom, about 2 more minutes.
4. Remove frittata to a plate.
5. In a small food processor, mix olives, tomatoes, chili flakes, and parsley. Blend until well chopped and blended, about 30 seconds.
6. Spread olive paste on top of frittata in an even layer.
7. Roll frittata into a tight roll, cut into 2 pieces and serve immediately.

SWEET FAT BOMBS

Cheesy Hazelnut Morsels

Prep time: 15 minutes

Cooking time: 0 minutes

Servings: 16

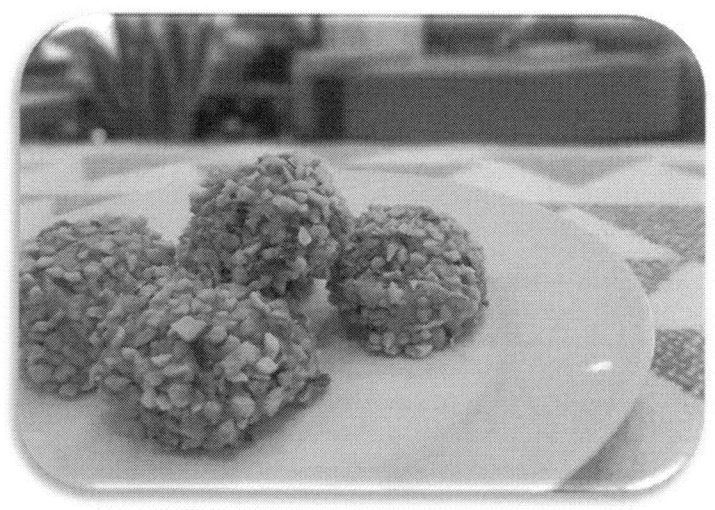

Nutrients per serving:

Carbohydrates – 3.4 g

Net Carbs – 1.2 g

Fat – 11.6 g

Protein – 3.2 g

Calories – 122

Ingredients:

- ½ cup ground hazelnuts
- ¼ cup hazelnut butter
- 1 cup cream cheese, softened
- ¼ cup cocoa powder
- 2 Tbsp sugar-free hazelnut syrup

Instructions:

1. Combine all ingredients except the ground hazelnuts.
2. Roll the cream cheese mixture into 16 balls.Place the ground hazelnuts in a bowl. Dip each ball into the ground hazelnuts.
3. Refrigerate for at least 2-3 hours.

Choco Mint Hazelnut Sticks

Prep time: 20 minutes

Cooking time: 0 minutes

Servings: 12

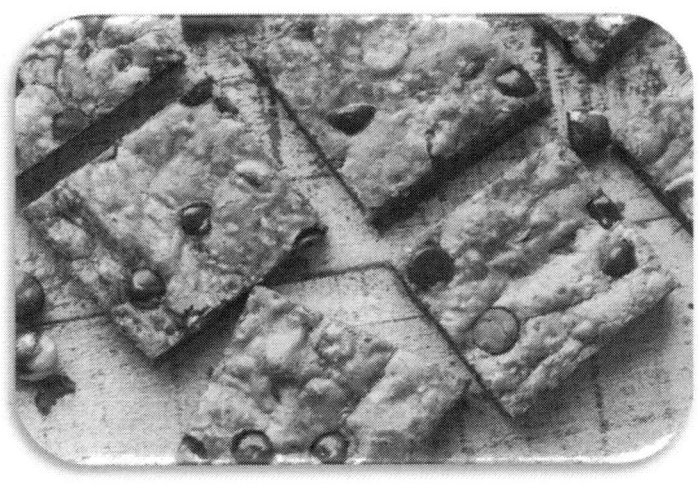

Nutrients per serving:

Carbohydrates – 5.6 g

Net Carbs – 2.4 g

Fat – 17 g

Protein – 3 g

Calories – 174

Ingredients:

- 4 Tbsp cocoa powder
- 1 cup shredded coconut
- 1 cup hazelnuts
- 1 tsp peppermint extract
- 6 Tbsp coconut oil, melted
- 4 Tbsp almond butter
- ¾ cup Stevia sweetener
- 1 tsp vanilla extract
- Salt, to taste

Instructions:

1. In a bowl, stir together the coconut oil, cacao powder, almond butter, sweetener, vanilla, peppermint extract, and salt. In a food processor, roughly chop the hazelnuts.
2. Heat the mixture slowly on low heat in a double boiler for 5 to 10 minutes until all ingredients are well combined.
3. Add hazelnuts and shredded coconut to the melted chocolate mixture and stir together.
4. Pour in a dish lined with parchment paper and freeze until chocolate is set, then cut into sticks.

Chocolate Keto Bomb

Prep time: 10 minutes

Cooking time: 0 minutes

Servings: 12

Nutrients per serving:

Carbohydrates – 2.55 g

Net Carbs – 0.71 g

Fat – 14.47 g

Protein – 1 g

Calories – 138

Ingredients:

- 1 Tbsp cacao powder
- 2 Tbsp chocolate protein powder
- 4 Tbsp coconut milk
- 2 Tbsp coconut flour
- 2 Tbsp coconut, shredded
- 1 Tbsp cacao nibs
- 1 tsp coconut oil, softened
- 2/3 cup coconut butter, softened

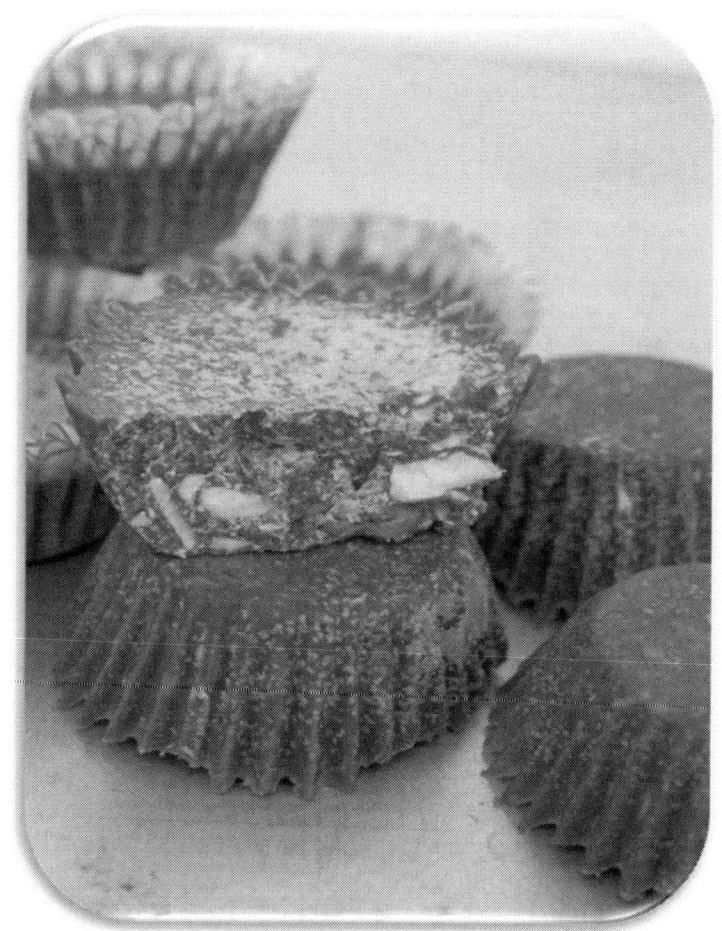

Instructions:

1. In a bowl, combine all ingredients except coconut oil with coconut butter. Whisk 2-3 minutes until well combined.
2. Spoon mixture into silicone molds.
3. Refrigirate for 30 minutes.
4. In a bowl, mix coconut oil with coconut butter. Remove molds from the refrigerator and cover with coating
5. Place back in the refrigerator until coating has hardened, about 1 hour.

Chocolate Peanut Butter Balls

Prep time: 10 minutes

Cooking time: 0 minutes

Servings: 12

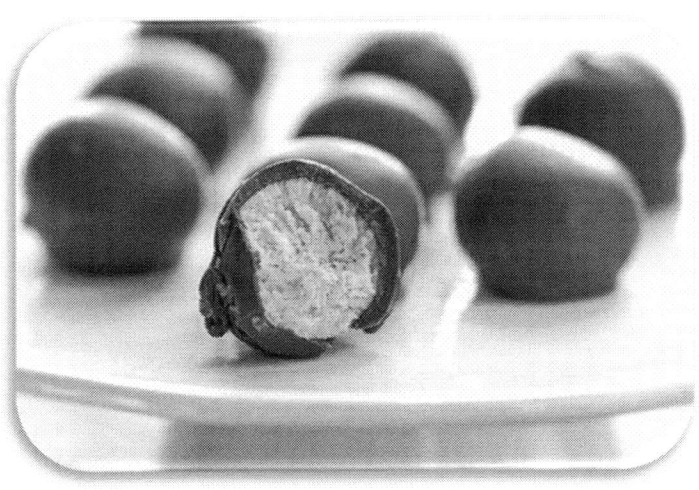

Nutrients per serving:

Carbohydrates – 5.16 g

Net Carbs – 2.54 g

Fat – 12 g

Protein – 3 g

Calories – 126

Ingredients:

- ½ stick butter, softened
- ½ cup natural peanut butter
- 2 Tbsp coconut flour
- 2 Tbsp vanilla whey protein powder
- ½ cup broken up sugar-free chocolate bars, melted
- 1 tsp organic vanilla extract
- 1½ cup powdered Xylitol

Instructions:

1. In a bowl, mix peanut butter and butter with electric hand mixer until smooth.
2. Add vanilla extract and protein, mix well.
3. Add powdered Xylitol sweetener and mix well.
4. Roll the dough into 24 bite sized balls. Place balls on a pan lined with a parchment paper.
5. Coat each ball with chocolate. Refrigerate for at least 2 hours.

Choco-Orange Walnut Muffin Bombs

Prep time: 20 minutes

Cooking time: 0 minutes

Servings: 18

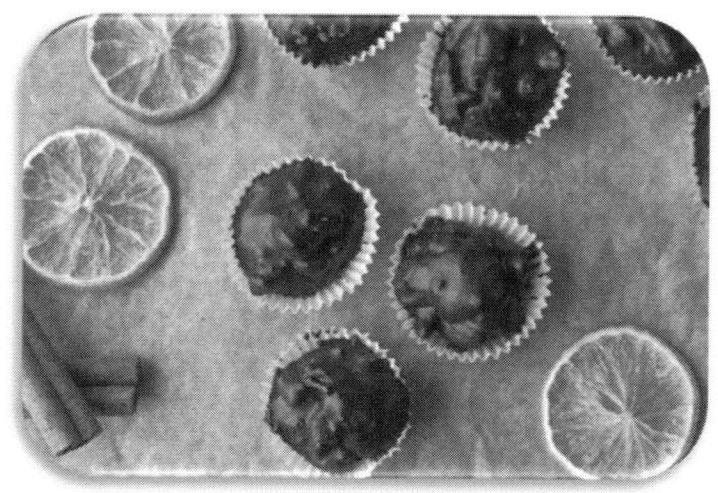

Nutrients per serving:

Carbohydrates – 5 g

Net Carbs – 3 g

Fat – 13 g

Protein – 13 g

Calories – 131

Ingredients:

- 1½ cup walnuts, chopped
- 4.40 oz dark chocolate, 100% cocoa
- 1 tsp natural orange extract
- 1 tsp fresh orange peel
- 4 Tbsp extra virgin coconut oil
- 15-20 drops of liquid Stevia
- 1 tsp cinnamon

Instructions:

1. Melt the chocolate using a double boiler. Add liquid Stevia, coconut oil, and cinnamon. Mix well.
2. Add fresh orange peel and natural orange extract. Add chopped walnuts and mix well.
3. Teaspoon mixture into small paper muffin cups.
4. Place in the fridge until solid, at least 4-6 hours.

Cinnamon Storm Fat Bombs

Prep time: 1 hour 30 minutes

Cooking time: 0 minutes

Servings: 12

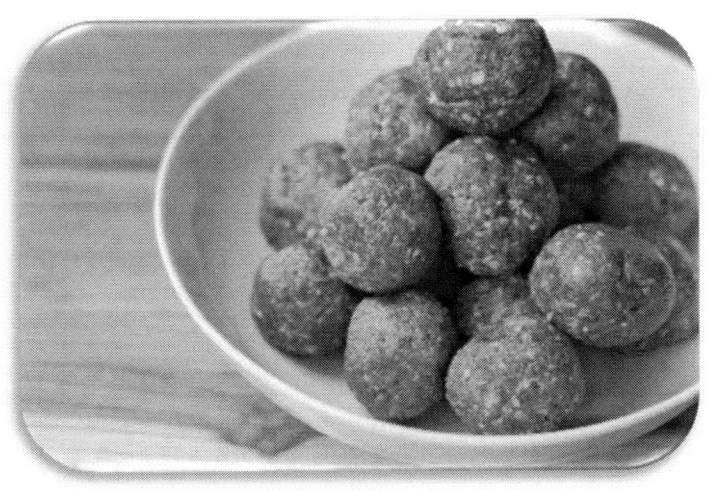

Nutrients per serving:

Carbohydrates – 1.6 g

Net Carbs – 0.2 g

Fat – 20 g

Protein – 1 g

Calories – 184

Ingredients:

- 1 cup coconut milk
- 1 cup almond butter
- 1 tsp pure vanilla extract
- ¾ tsp cinnamon
- ½ tsp nutmeg
- 1 tsp natural sweetener, to your taste
- 1 cup coconut shreds

Instructions:

1. Add all ingredients except shredded coconut in a double boiler. Stir constantly to melt and combine well.
2. When ready, remove from the heat. Let cool for 5-6 minutes. Refrigirate for 45 minutes, until hard.
3. Put the coconut shreds in a bowl. Roll the coconut-cinnamon mixture into one inch balls and roll them through the coconut shreds.
4. Place the balls on a serving plate and refrigerate for 2-3 hours.

Frozen Maca-Nutty Bites

Prep time: 2 hours 15 minutes

Cooking time: 0 minutes

Servings: 12

Nutrients per serving:

Carbohydrates – 2 g

Net Carbs – 0.65 g

Fat – 9 g

Protein – 2 g

Calories – 93

Ingredients:

- ¼ cup coconut oil
- ¼ cup almond butter
- 1 tsp vanilla extract
- 12 drops liquid stevia
- 2 Tbsp cocoa powder
- 12 whole macadamia nuts

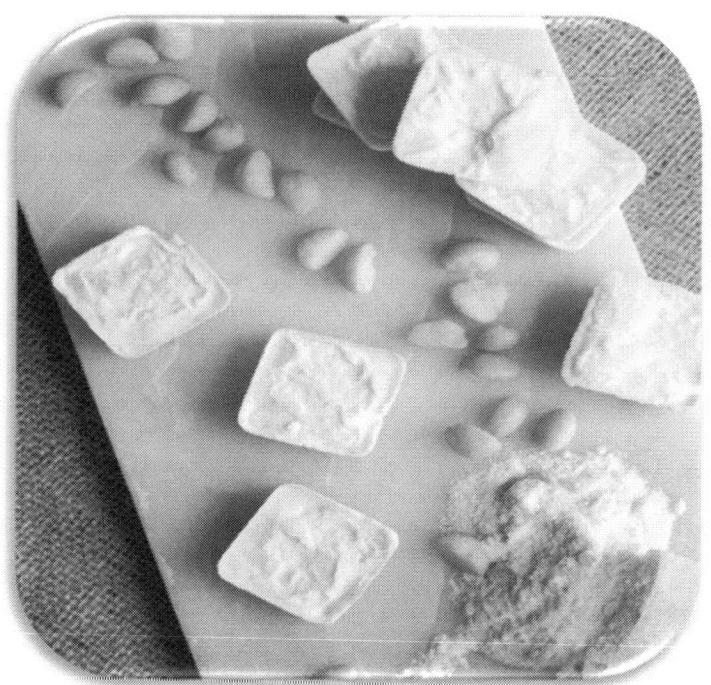

Instructions:

1. Combine coconut oil, almond butter, vanilla, and stevia in a small saucepan over medium heat, frequently stirring until ingredients have melted. Turn off heat.
2. Add cocoa powder and stir well to combine.
3. Pour mixture into 12 molds of a silicone ice cube tray or silicone candy mold tray until about half full.
4. Place 1 macadamia nut into each filled mold.
5. Freeze until set. Serve from the freezer.

Keto Orange Fat Bites

Prep time: 10 minutes

Cooking time: 0 minutes

Servings: 14

Nutrients per serving:

Carbohydrates – 0.5 g

Net Carbs – 0.2 g

Fat – 14 g

Protein – 1 g

Calories – 127

Ingredients:

- ½ cup heavy whipping cream
- ½ cup cream cheese
- ½ cup coconut oil, melted
- 1 tsp pure orange extract
- 10 drops Liquid Stevia

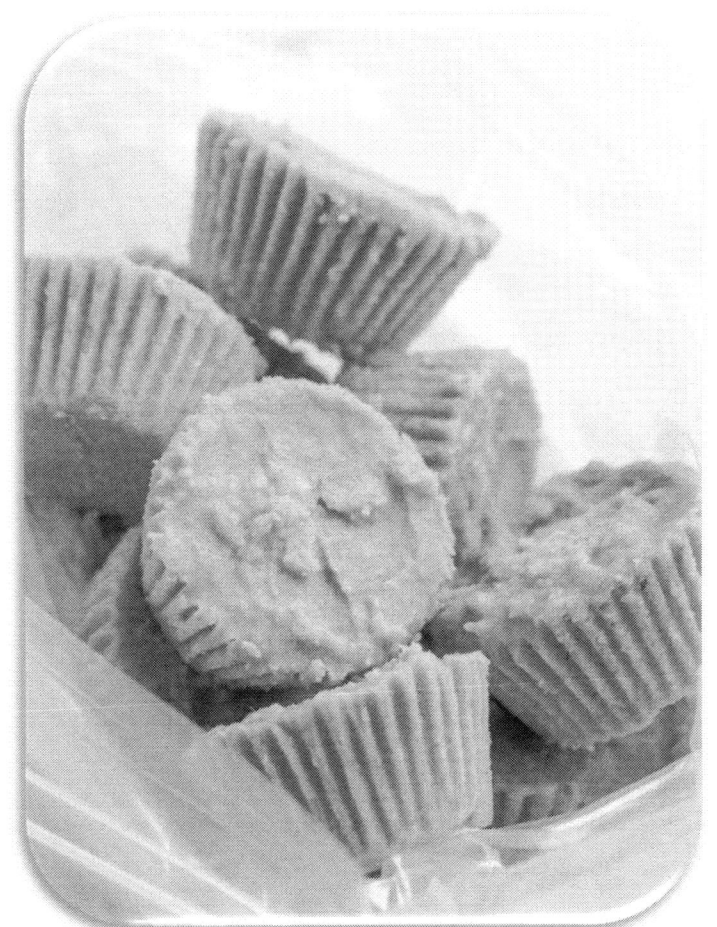

Instructions:

1. Blend all ingredients together.
2. Spoon the batter into a silicone tray or paper muffin cups.
3. Refrigerate for 2 hours. Before serving remove from silicone tray and serve. Keep refrigerated.

Easy Choco Blueberry Fat Bombs

Prep time: 15 minutes

Cooking time: 0 minutes

Servings: 6

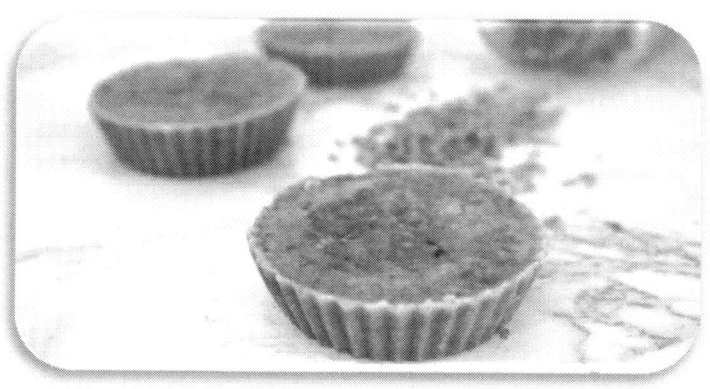

Nutrients per serving:

Carbohydrates – 1 g

Net Carbs – 0.05 g

Fat – 17 g

Protein – 0.5 g

Calories – 148

Ingredients:

- 5 Tbsp butter
- 3 Tbsp coconut oil
- 2 Tbsp sugar-free Blueberry syrup
- 2 Tbsp cocoa powder

Instructions:

1. In a saucepan, cook all ingredients over low heat until well combined.
2. Transfer into a silicone mold and freeze for at least 3 hours.

Easy Cream Cheese Jello Balls

Prep time: 10 minutes

Cooking time: 0 minutes

Servings: 8

Nutrients per serving:

Carbohydrates – 1.2 g

Net Carbs – 1 g

Fat – 16 g

Protein – 2 g

Calories – 150

Ingredients:

- 1 cup cream cheese
- ¼ cup coconut butter
- 1 package of sugar-free jello

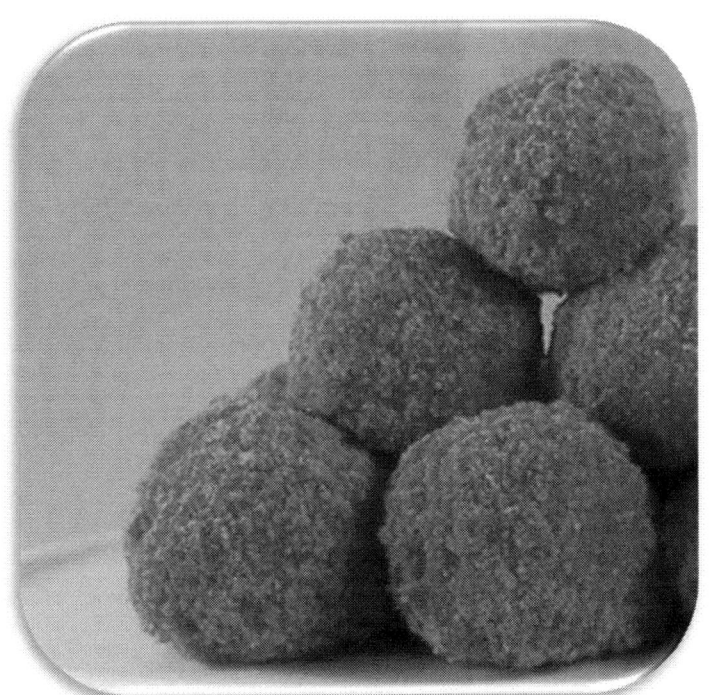

Instructions:

1. Put jello powder in small bowl.
2. In a bowl, combine cream cheese and coconut butter.
3. Take a teaspoon of cream cheese mixture and roll into a ball in your hands and then roll in the jello powder. Make 16 balls.
4. Cover with plastic wrap and refrigirate for 2 hours.

Gingery Coconut Fat Bomb

Prep time: 5 minutes

Cooking time: 0 minutes

Servings: 10

Nutrients per serving:

Carbohydrates – 2.5 g

Net Carbs – 0.3 g

Fat – 14.5 g

Protein – 2 g

Calories – 134

Ingredients:

- 1 tsp ginger, dried, powdered
- 0.8 oz shredded coconut
- 1/3 cup coconut oil, softened
- 1/3 cup coconut butter, softened
- 1 tsp granulated sweetener of choice, to taste

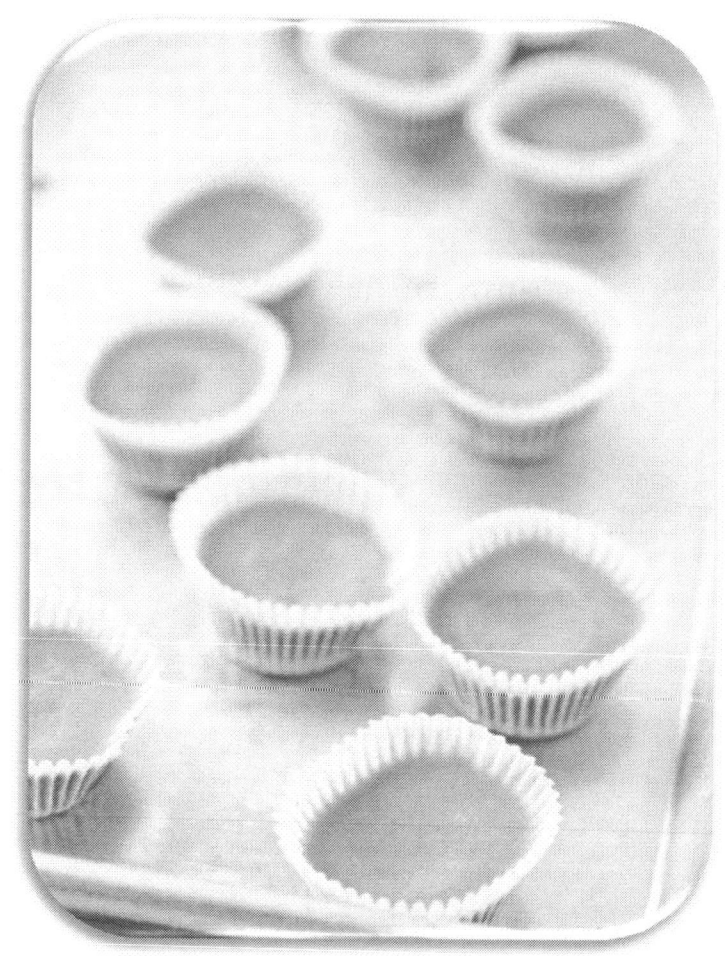

Instructions:

1. Combine all ingredients until well mixed.
2. Pour the ginger mixture into paper muffin cups and refrigerate for 1 hour to solidify.

Homemade Keto Almond Butter

Prep time: 25 minutes

Cooking time: 12 minutes

Servings: 14

Nutrients per serving:

Carbohydrates – 5.5 g

Net Carbs – 1.3 g

Fat – 13.5 g

Protein – 5 g

Calories – 153

Ingredients:

- 3 cups almonds, no salt added
- 1 tsp Himalayan salt
- 1 tsp cinnamon
- 1 vanilla pod or bean, halved, seeds removed
- 2 Tbsp Stevia powder or Erythritol sweetener

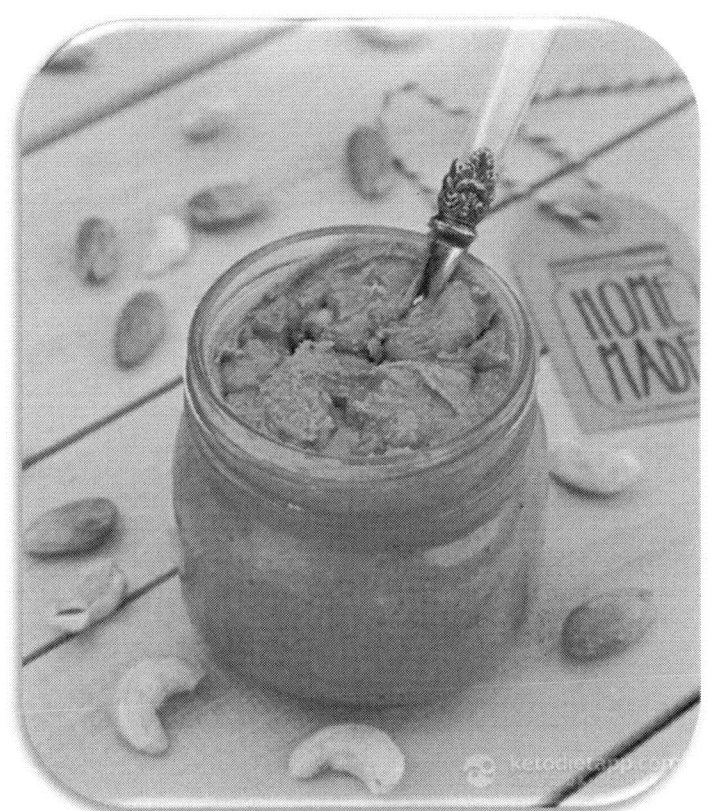

Instructions:

1. Preheat oven to 360°F. Place almonds in a baking pan and bake for 10-12 minutes. Stir occasionally not to burn.
2. Add the almonds and remaining ingredients to a food processor.
3. Process for 15 minutes above. Pour the almond butter into a glass container and store in the refrigerator.

Keto Almond Cookies Bombs

Prep time: 25 minutes

Cooking time: 18 minutes

Servings: 16

Nutrients per serving:

Carbohydrates – 3.35 g

Net Carbs – 0.5 g

Fat – 17 g

Protein – 2.9 g

Calories – 171

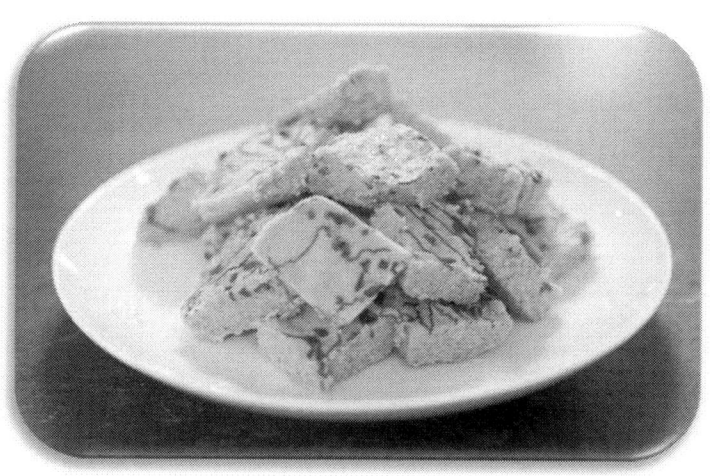

Ingredients:

- 1 cup almonds, chopped
- 1 cup butter, softened
- 2 ¼ cups almond flour
- 1¼ cup cocoa powder
- 3½ Tbsp coconut flour
- 2 eggs
- ¾ cup Stevia powder
- 2 tsp vanilla extract
- ½ tsp baking soda
- ¼ tsp sea salt

Instructions:

1. Preheat oven to 340°F.
2. In a bowl, whisk butter and sweetener. Stir in the eggs, coconut oil, and vanilla extract.
3. In a separate bowl, mix together the baking soda, almond flour, coconut flour, cocoa powder, and salt.
4. Combine the eggs mixture to the flour mixture. Pour dough into a greased baking pan. Sprinkle dough with chopped almond.
5. Bake for 15-18 minutes. Let cool and cut into chunks. Serve.

Keto Hazelnuts Fat Bomb Squares

Prep time: 2 hours 15 minutes

Cooking time: 0 minutes

Servings: 6

Nutrients per serving:

Carbohydrates – 3.8 g

Net Carbs – 0.5 g

Fat – 16.5 g

Protein – 2 g

Calories – 160

Ingredients:

- ½ cup hazelnuts, chopped
- 1 cup whipped cream
- ¼ cup cocoa butter
- 2 Tbs cocoa powder, unsweetened
- 2 Tbs Stevia sweetener

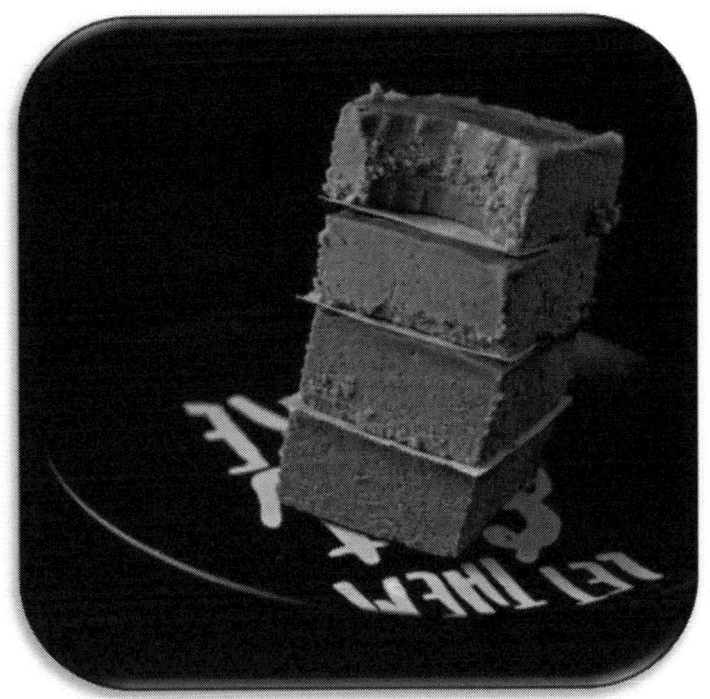

Instructions:

1. In a bowl, melt cocoa butter at room temperature.
2. When ready, add in cocoa powder and Stevia powder. Mix until all ingredients are well blended. Add in chopped hazelnuts and stir well.
3. Finally, add whipping cream and mix well.
4. Pour the hazelnut mixture in squared molds or ice cube trays and refrigerate for 1-2 hours.

Keto Lime Fat Bombs

Prep time: 2 hours 10 minutes

Cooking time: 0 minutes

Servings: 16

Nutrients per serving:

Carbohydrates – 0.9 g

Net Carbs – 0.15 g

Fat – 12.5 g

Protein – 0.2 g

Calories – 109

Ingredients:

- 2 limes zest
- 1 cup extra-virgin coconut oil, softened
- ¾ cup coconut butter, softened
- 20 drops Erythritol extract
- Salt, to taste

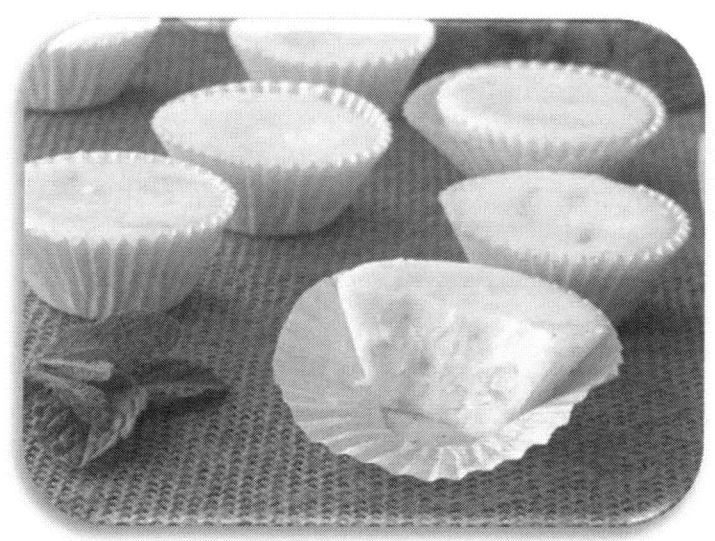

Instructions:

1. Soften the coconut butter and coconut oil at room temperature.
2. In a bowl, mix all ingredients.
3. Spoon mixture into 16 mini muffin cups.
4. Refrigerate for 2 hours.

Lemon Coconut Fat Bombs

Prep time: 4 hours 15 minutes

Cooking time: 0 minutes

Servings: 12

Nutrients per serving:

Carbohydrates – 1 g

Net Carbs – 0.8 g

Fat – 12 g

Protein – 1.3 g

Calories – 106

Ingredients:

- ¼ cup shredded coconut, unsweetened,
- 1 cup cream cheese
- 1 Tbsp pure lemon extract
- Natural sweetener of your choice, to taste
- ¼ cup butter

Instructions:

1. In a bowl, combine cream cheese, natural sweetener, and lemon extract. Place bowl in refrigerator for 15-20 minutes.
2. In a separate bowl, add unsweetened shredded coconut.

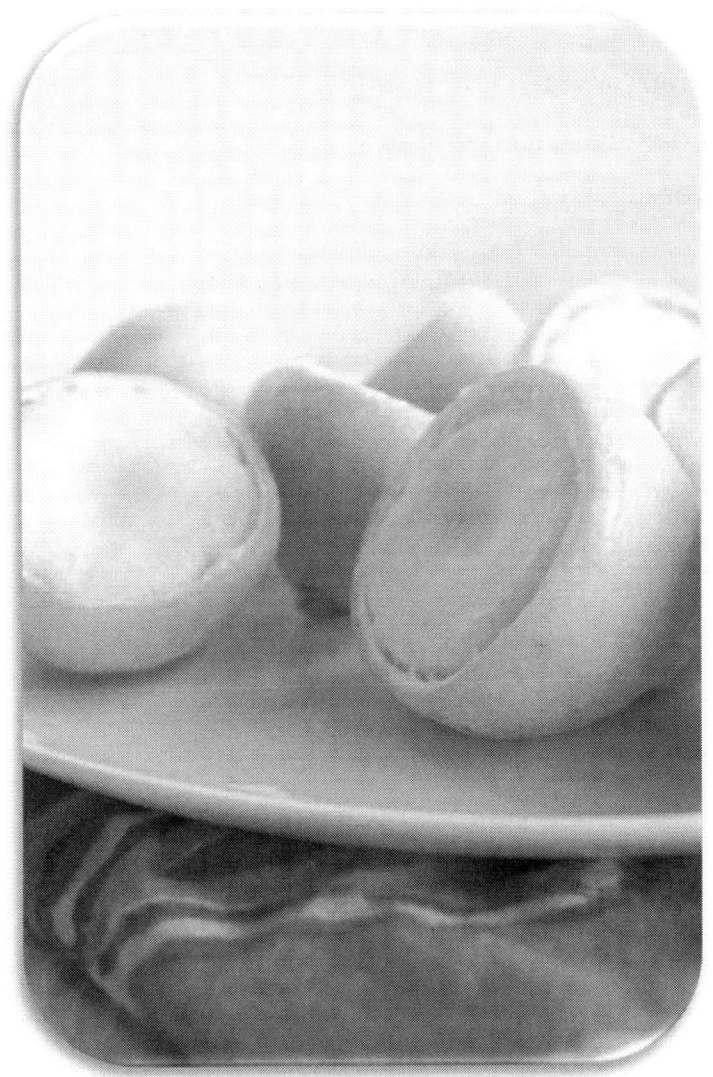

3. Roll lemon batter into 16 equal balls. Dip each ball into coconut and place on a serving pan. Refrigerate for 3-4 hours. Serve.

Lemony Cream Cheese Bombshells

Prep time: 2 hours 10 minutes

Cooking time: 0 minutes

Servings: 12

Nutrients per serving:

Carbohydrates – 0.8 g

Net Carbs – 0.7 g

Fat – 14.5 g

Protein – 1.3 g

Calories – 134

Ingredients:

- ½ cup unsalted butter, softened
- 1 cup cream cheese, softened
- ½ tsp pure lemon extract
- ¾ cup granular Stevia

Instructions:

1. Combine all ingredients with an electric mixer for several minutes, until soft.
2. Place teaspoons of mixture on a wax paper-lined sheet.

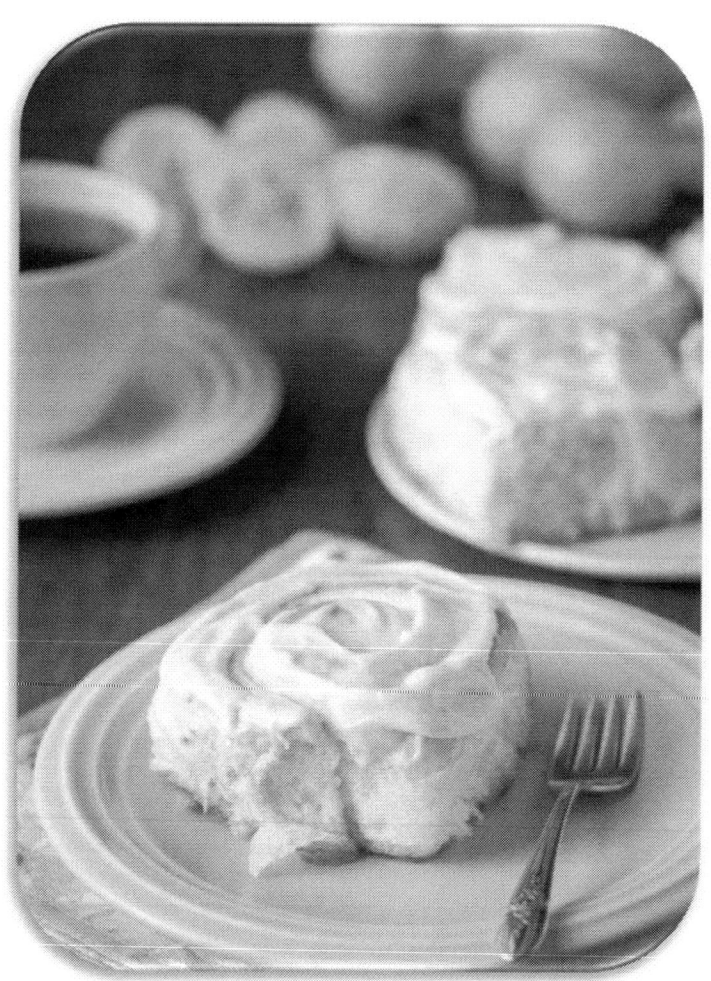

3. Freeze until firm, at least 2 hours. Remove to the freezer and serve frozen.

Heavenly Lemon Quads with Coconut Cream

Prep time: 6 hours 15 minutes

Cooking time: 35 minutes

Servings: 8

Nutrients per serving:

Carbohydrates – 4 g

Net Carbs – 1.4 g

Fat – 15 g

Protein – 5 g

Calories – 129

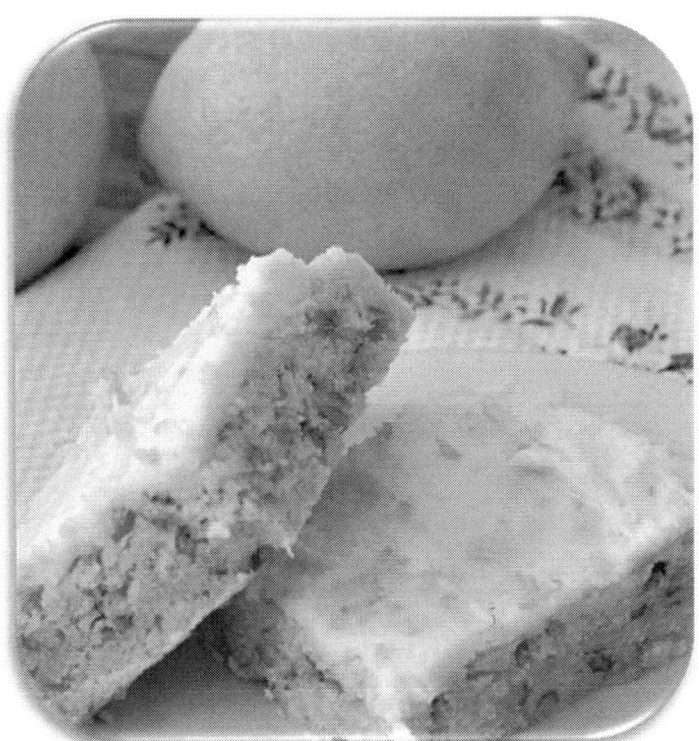

Ingredients:

- ¾ cup coconut flakes
- 2 Tbsp coconut oil
- 1 Tbsp ground almonds
- 5 eggs
- ½ lemon juice
- 1 Tbsp coconut flour
- ½ cup Stevia sweetener

Instructions:

1. Preheat oven to 360°F.
2. In a bowl, putcoconut flakes, coconut oil, ground almonds, and mix everything until soft.
3. With coconut oil, grease a rectanglular oven dish. Pour dough in a dish and bake for 15 minutes until golden brown. Set aside to cool.
4. In a bowl, whisk together eggs, lemon juice, coconut flour, and sweetener. Pour over the baked cake evenly.
5. Bake 20 minutes more.
6. Set aside for a few minutes and then refrigerate for at least 6 hours.

Frozen Butter Rum Chocolate

Prep time: 3 hours 15 minutes

Cooking time: 0 minutes

Servings: 12

Nutrients per serving:

Carbohydrates – 2 g

Net Carbs – 0.47 g

Fat – 7 g

Protein – 2 g

Calories – 75

Ingredients:

- ¼ cup coconut oil
- ¼ cup almond butter
- 2 tsp rum extract
- 12 drops liquid stevia
- 2 Tbsp cocoa powder

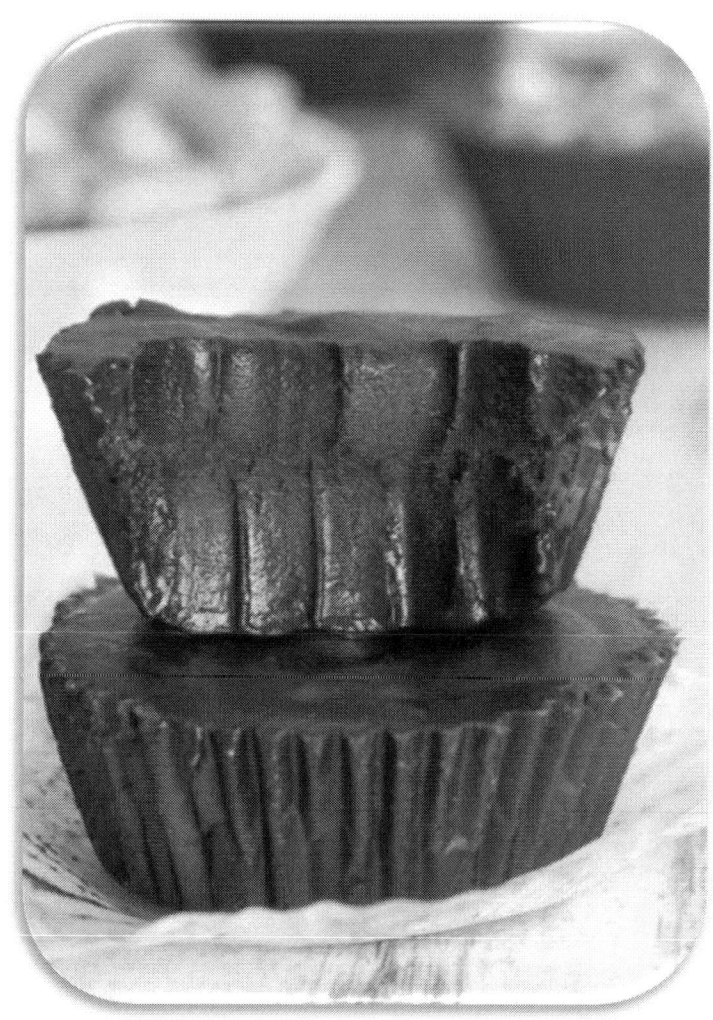

Instructions:

1. Mix all ingredients except cocoa powder in a small saucepan over medium heat, frequently stirring until ingredients have melted. Turn off heat.
2. Add cocoa powder and stir well to combine.
3. Pour mixture into 12 molds of a silicone-bottomed ice cube tray or silicone candy mold tray.
4. Freeze until set. Serve from the freezer.

Macadamia Cacao Fat Bombs

Prep time: 6 hours 10 minutes

Cooking time: 0 minutes

Servings: 24

Nutrients per serving:

Carbohydrates – 7 g

Net Carbs – 3.4 g

Fat – 13 g

Protein – 3.5 g

Calories – 143

Ingredients:

- 1 cup macadamia nuts, chopped
- ½ cup cacao powder
- 2 cups almond flour
- ½ cup ground flax
- 3 Tbsp coconut oil, melted
- 1/3 cup Stevia
- 1/3 cup water
- ½ tsp pure vanilla extract

Instructions:

1. In a bowl, mix almond flour, flax, and cacao powder. Stir in oil, water, sweetener, and vanilla. Then stir in chopped hazelnuts.

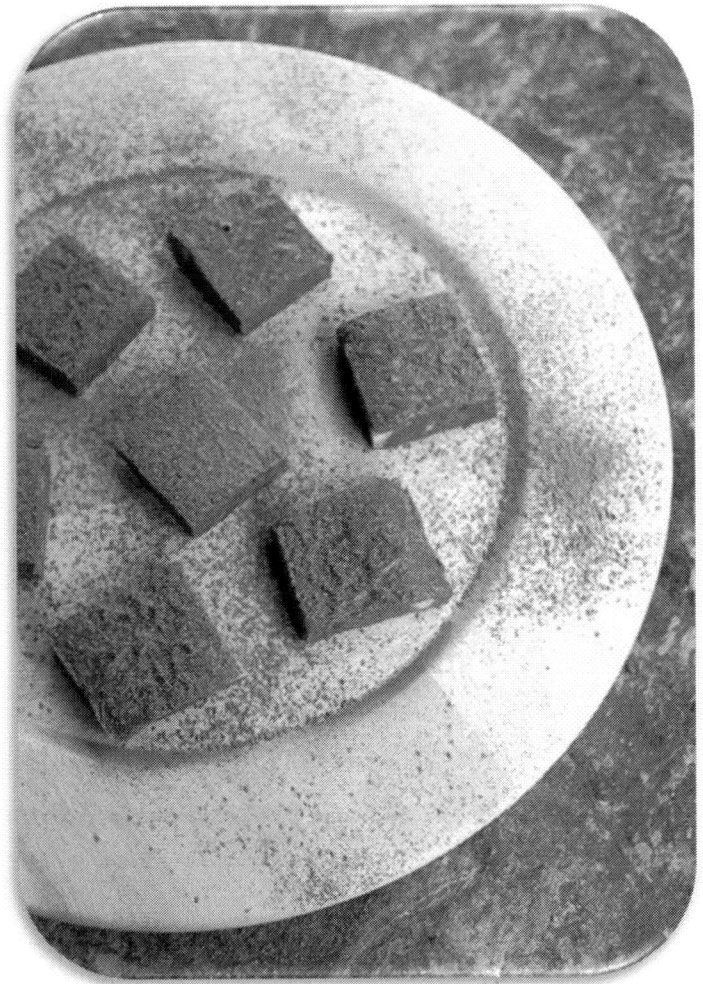

2. Create balls out from the mixture, press flat with palms, and place on dehydrator screens.

3. Dehydrate for 1 hour at 145°. Reduce to 116° and dehydrate for about 5 hours until desired dryness is achieved.

Minty Keto Galettes

Prep time: 4 hours 20 minutes

Cooking time: 0 minutes

Servings: 18

Nutrients per serving:

Carbohydrates – 0.5 g

Net Carbs – 0.1 g

Fat – 11 g

Protein – 0.25 g

Calories – 93

Ingredients:

- 3 cup coconut butter, melted
- 1 cup coconut, shredded
- 3 Tbsp coconut oil melted
- ¾ tsp pure peppermint extract
- 2 Tbsp cacao powder

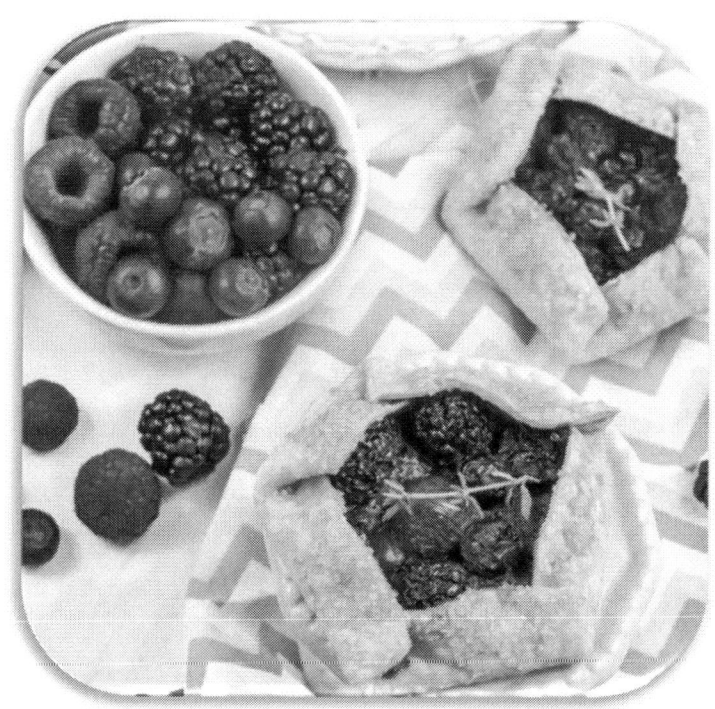

Instructions:

1. In a bowl, combine 1 Tbsp of coconut oil and 3/4 tsp peppermint extract, shredded coconut and melted coconut butter.
2. Fill mini muffin tins halfway with coconut butter. Put in refrigerator for about 20 minutes.
3. In a separate bowl, combine 2 Tbsp coconut oil and cacao powder.
4. Pour mixture on top of chilled cocount butter.
5. Return to refrigerator for 3-4 hours. Serve.

Peanut Butter Candy with Chocolate Sauce

Prep time: 3 hours 10 minutes

Cooking time: 0 minutes

Servings: 12

Nutrients per serving:

Carbohydrates – 5.8 g

Net Carbs – 2.4 g

Fat – 27 g

Protein – 6 g

Calories – 273

Ingredients:

- 1 cup peanut butter
- ¼ cup almond milk, unsweetened
- 1 cup coconut oil
- 2 tsp liquid Stevia sweetener
- Chocolate Sauce Topping
- 2 Tbsp coconut oil, melted
- 4 Tbsp cocoa powder, unsweetened
- 2 Tbsp Stevia sweetener

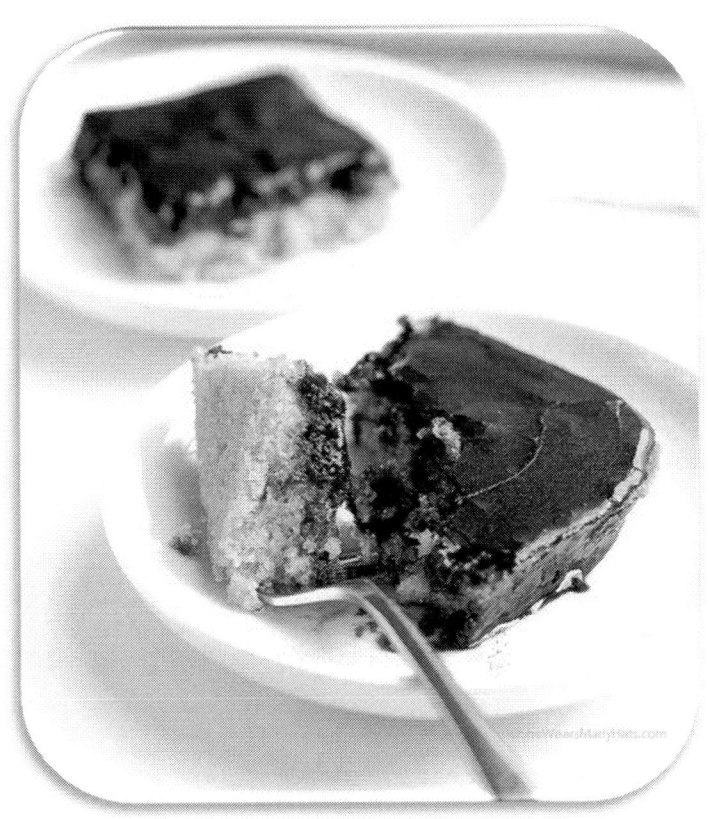

Instructions:

1. In a microwave-safe bowl, mix coconut oil and peanut butter; melt in microwave for 1-2 minutes.
2. Blend this mixture with the rest of the ingredients until combined.
3. Pour the peanut mixture into a parchment lined loaf pan or platter.
4. Refrigerate for about 3 hours.
5. In a bowl, whisk all topping ingredients together. Pour over the peanut candy.

Peppermint Fat Bombs

Prep time: 2 hours 10 minutes

Cooking time: 0 minutes

Servings: 25

Nutrients per serving:

Carbohydrates – 8 g

Net Carbs – 0.25 g

Fat – 19 g

Protein – 22 g

Calories – 202

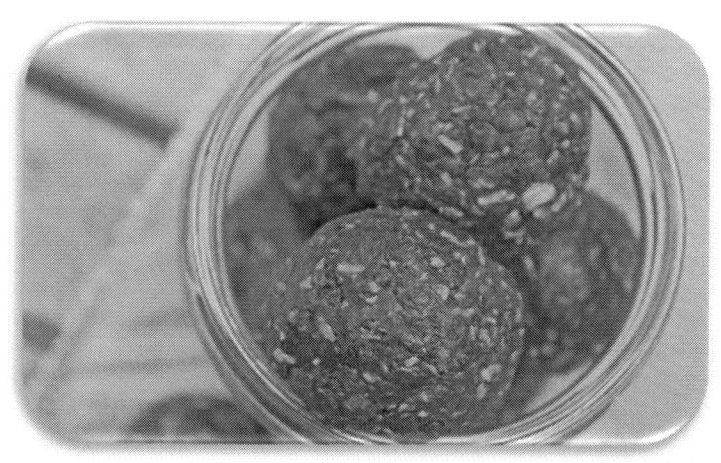

Ingredients:

- 1¼ cup seed butter
- 1 tsp peppermint extract
- 1½ cups coconut oil
- ½ cup sweetener (liquid or granulated)
- 2 tsp organic vanilla extract
- ¼ tsp salt

Instructions:

1. Melt the coconut oil.
2. Blend all ingredients until smooth.
3. Make 25 coconut balls from the mixture.
4. Freeze the balls on a baking sheet until solid. Keep refrigerated.

Pistachio Masala Fat Bombs

Prep time: 5 hours 15 minutes

Cooking time: 0 minutes

Servings: 32

Nutrients per serving:

Carbohydrates – 0.4 g

Net Carbs – 0.1 g

Fat – 17 g

Protein – 0.27 g

Calories – 147

Ingredients:

- 1 cup almond butter, melted
- ¼ cup ghee
- 1 cup coconut oil
- ½ cup cocoa butter
- ¼ cup pistachio nuts
- 1 Tbs coconut milk
- 1 Tbsp pure vanilla extract
- 2 tsp Masala chai

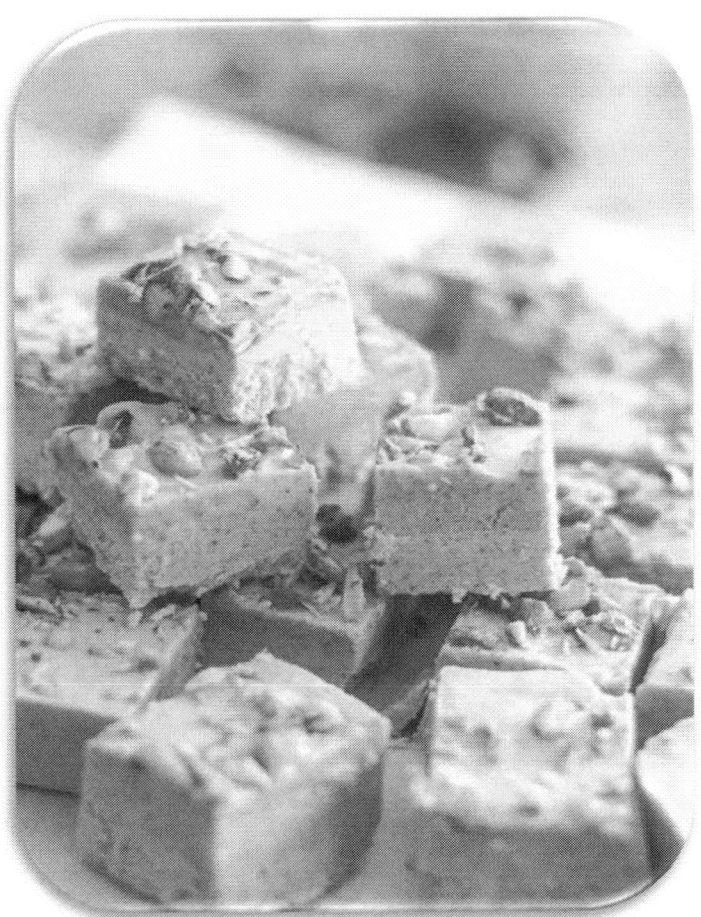

Instructions:

1. In a saucepan, melt the cocoa butter over low heat.
2. In a large bowl, combine all ingredients with a hand mixer, except cocoa butter and pistachios.
3. Add in the melted butter and blend for 1-2 minutes more.
4. Transfer the mixture to greased and paper-lined pan. Sprinkle with chopped pistachios and refrigerate for at least 5 hours.

Raspberry Heaven Fat Bombs

Prep time: 2 hours 20 minutes

Cooking time: 0 minutes

Servings: 18

Nutrients per serving:

Carbohydrates – 0.6 g

Net Carbs – 0.4 g

Fat – 12 g

Protein – 0.77 g

Calories – 101

Ingredients:

- 3 Tbsp heavy cream
- ¼ cup coconut oil, melted
- 8 oz cream cheese, softened
- ¼ cup coconut oil, melted
- 3 tsp raspberry extract
- ½ cup powdered Erythritol
- Salt, to taste
- 5 drops natural red food coloring

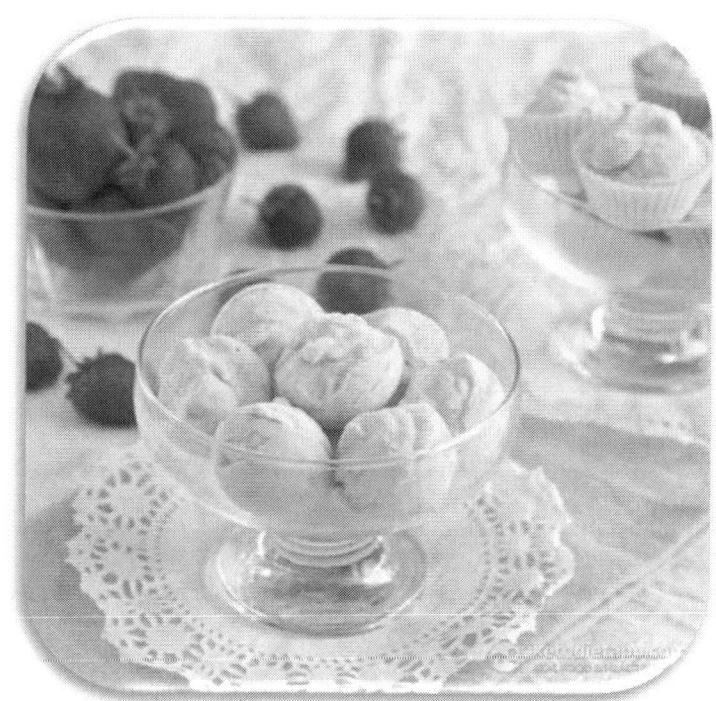

Instructions:

1. Blend the cream cheese and sweetener together with a hand mixer.
2. Add the raspberry extract, natural food coloring, cream, salt, and raspberry extract and blend.
3. Add the coconut oil and continue to blend until it's smooth and creamy.
4. Refrigerate the mixture for 1 hour.
5. When ready, make 48 small balls from batter and place on a parchment-lined baking sheet. Place in the freezer for 2 hours.

Slow Cooker Pecan Nuts Fat Bomb

Prep time: 15 minutes

Cooking time: 2 hours 15 minutes

Servings: 8

Nutrients per serving:

Carbohydrates – 3.6 g

Net Carbs – 0.88 g

Fat – 14 g

Protein – 2.9 g

Calories – 140

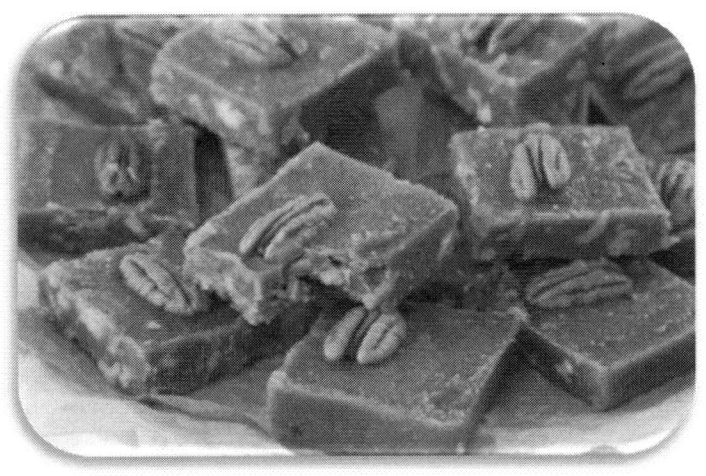

Ingredients:

- 2 cups Pecans nuts, halves
- 4 Tbsp almond butter
- 1 cup Stevia or any other natural sweetener
- ¼ tsp ground ginger
- ¼ tsp ground allspice
- 1½ tsp ground cinnamon

Instructions:

1. In a 4-quart Slow Cooker, stir the pecan halves and almond butter until combined.
2. Add Stevia and stir well.
3. Add spices and stir well to coat.
4. Cook on high covered for 10 minutes. Turn to low and cook uncovered for about 2 hours, or until the nuts are a little crispy.

Lemonade Fat Bomb

Prep time: 2 hours 10 minutes

Cooking time: 0 minutes

Servings: 2

Nutrients per serving:

Carbohydrates – 8 g

Net Carbs – 4 g

Fat – 43 g

Protein – 4 g

Calories – 404

Ingredients:

- ½ lemon
- 4 oz cream cheese, at room temperature
- 2 oz butter, at room temperature
- 2 tsp Swerve natural sweetener or
- 2 drops liquid stevia
- Pinch pink salt

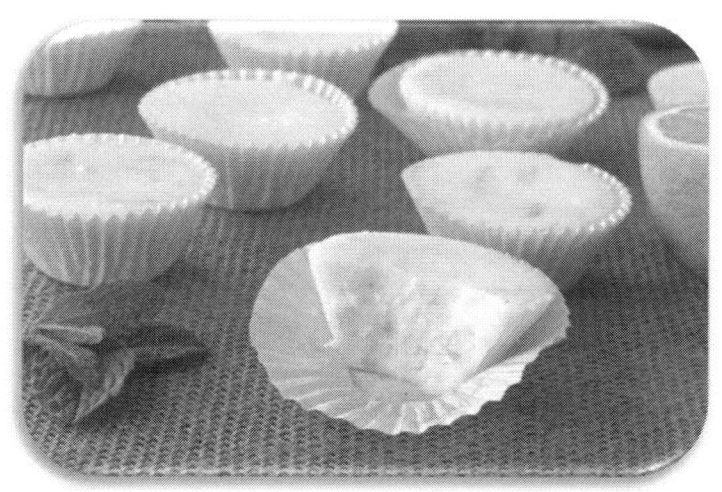

Instructions:

1. Zest the lemon, squeeze the juice from the lemon half into the bowl with the zest.
2. Combine the cream cheese and butter. Add the sweetener, lemon zest and juice, and pink salt. Beat with a hand mixer. until fully combined
3. Spoon the mixture into molds. Freeze for at least 2 hours.

Berry Cheesecake Fat Bomb

Prep time: 2 hours 10 minutes

Cooking time: 0 minutes

Servings: 2

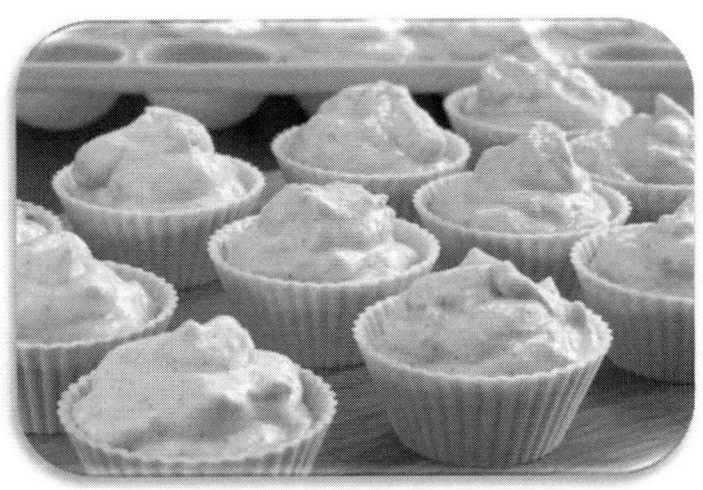

Nutrients per serving:

Carbohydrates – 9 g

Net Carbs – 4 g

Fat – 43 g

Protein – 4 g

Calories – 414

Ingredients:

- 4 oz cream cheese, room temperature
- 4 Tbsp butter, room temperature
- 2 tsp Swerve natural sweetener or 2 drops liquid stevia
- 1 tsp vanilla extract
- ¼ cup berries, fresh or frozen

Instructions:

1. With a hand mixer mix the cream cheese, butter, sweetener, and vanilla.
2. In a small bowl, mash the berries thoroughly. Add the berries into the cream cheese mixture using a rubber scraper.
3. Spoon the cream-cheese mixture into molds.
4. Freeze for at least 2 hours.

Crustless Cheesecake Bites

Prep time: 3 hours 10 minutes

Cooking time: 30 minutes

Servings: 2

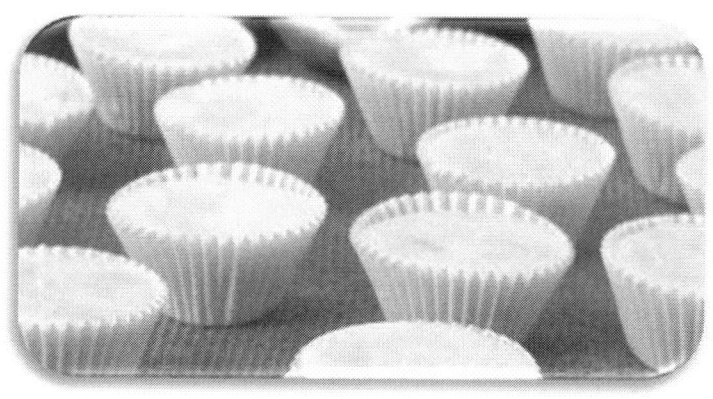

Nutrients per serving:

Carbohydrates – 18 g

Net Carbs – 2 g

Fat – 15 g

Protein – 5 g

Calories – 169

Ingredients:

- 4 oz cream cheese, at room temperature
- ¼ cup sour cream
- 2 large eggs
- ½ cup Swerve natural sweetener
- 1 tsp vanilla extract

Instructions:

1. Preheat oven to 350°F.
2. With a hand mixer beat the cream cheese, sour cream, eggs, sweetener, and vanilla until well mixed.
3. Place silicone liners (or cupcake paper liners) in the cups of a muffin tin.
4. Pour the cheesecake batter into the liners and bake for 30 minutes.
5. Refrigerate until completely cooled before serving, about 3 hours.

Pumpkin Crustless Cheesecake Bites

Prep time: 3 hours 10 minutes

Cooking time: 30 minutes

Servings: 4

Nutrients per serving:

Carbohydrates – 21 g

Net Carbs – 4 g

Fat – 12 g

Protein – 5 g

Calories – 156

Ingredients:

- 4 oz pumpkin purée
- 4 oz cream cheese, at room temperature
- 2 large eggs
- ½ cup Swerve natural sweetener
- 2 tsp pumpkin pie spice

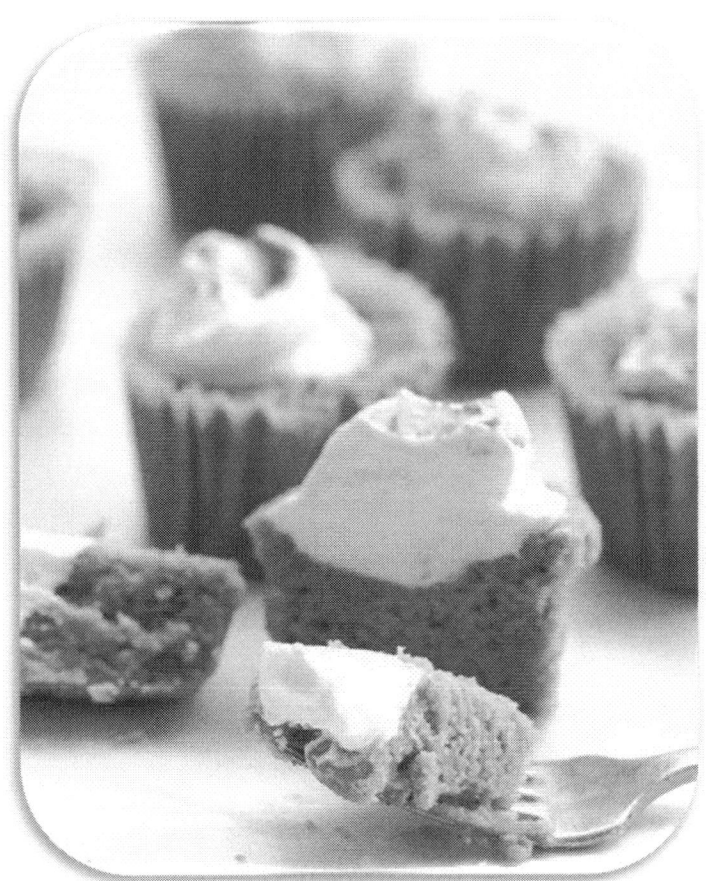

Instructions:

1. Preheat oven to 350°F.
2. With a hand mixer mix the pumpkin purée, cream cheese, eggs, sweetener, and pumpkin pie spice until thoroughly combined.
3. Place silicone liners or cupcake paper liners into the cups of a muffin tin.
4. Transfer the batter into the liners, and bake for 30 minutes.
5. Refrigerate until completely cooled before serving, about 3 hours.

Peppermint Fudge Fat Bomb

Prep time: 40 minutes

Cooking time: 0 minutes

Servings: 10

Nutrients per serving:

Carbohydrates – 1 g

Net Carbs – 0 g

Fat – 12 g

Protein – 0 g

Calories – 117

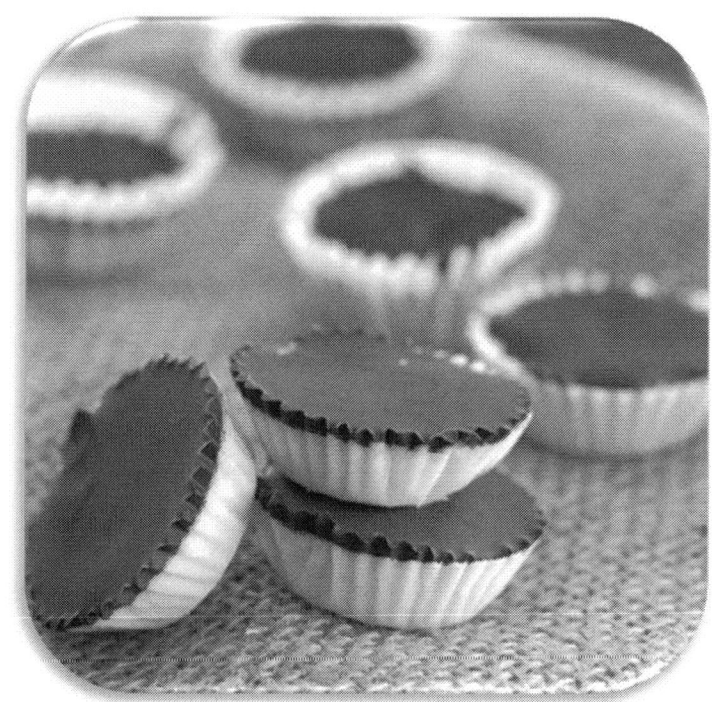

Ingredients:

- 1/3 cup coconut oil, melted
- 3 Tbsp sugar-free vanilla bean sweetener, divided
- 2 Tbsp organic heavy whipping cream, divided
- 1 tsp mint extract
- 2 Tbsp golden ghee
- 1 oz unsweetened chocolate

Instructions:

1. Line 10 cups of a 12-count mini-cupcake tin with parchment cups.
2. In a single-serving blender, combine the coconut oil, 2 Tbsp sweetener, 1 Tbsp heavy cream, and mint extract. Blend until thick, about 30 seconds. Pour the mixture into the cups, filling each half full. Place the tin in the freezer.
3. Meanwhile, combine the ghee and chocolate in a small microwave-safe bowl. Microwave on high in 15-second intervals for 2 minutes.
4. Stir in the remaining 1 Tbsp of sweetener and 1 Tbsp of heavy cream and mix until smooth.
5. Remove the cupcake tin from the freezer. Fill the cups with the chocolate mixture.Freeze for at least 30 minutes. Store in an airtight container in the freezer or refrigerator.

Peanut Butter Fudge Fat Squares

Prep time: 40 minutes

Cooking time: 0 minutes

Servings: 10

Nutrients per serving:

Carbohydrates – 2 g

Net Carbs – 1 g

Fat – 10 g

Protein – 2 g

Calories – 102

Ingredients:

- ¼ cup smooth peanut butter
- 4 Tbsp golden ghee, divided
- 1½ Tbsp sugar-free vanilla bean sweetener, divided
- 1 oz unsweetened chocolate
- 1 Tbsp organic heavy cream

Instructions:

1. Line 10 cups of a 12-count mini-cupcake tin with parchment cups.
2. In a small bowl, mix the peanut butter, 2 Tbsp of ghee, and ½ Tbsp of sweetener until smooth. Pour the mixture into the mini-cupcake cups, filling each half full. Place the tin in the freezer.

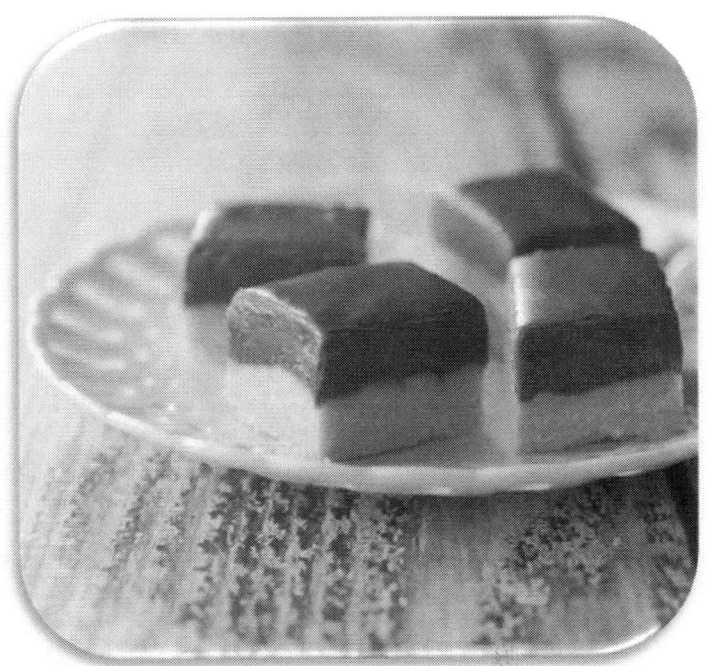

3. In a microwave-safe bowl, add the remaining 2 Tbsp of ghee and the chocolate. Microwave on high in 15-second intervals, stirring after each, for 2 minutes until the chocolate becomes soft and mixes easily with the ghee.
4. Stir in the remaining 1 Tbsp of sweetener and the heavy cream and mix until smooth.
5. Remove the cupcake tin from the freezer. Fill each cup with the chocolate mixture. Return the tin to the freezer to chill for at least 30 minutes. Store in a refrigerator.

Peanut Butter-Avocado Fat Bombs

Prep time: 3 hours 10 minutes

Cooking time: 0 minutes

Servings: 6

Nutrients per serving:

Carbohydrates – 9 g

Net Carbs – 4 g

Fat – 68 g

Protein – 12 g

Calories – 653

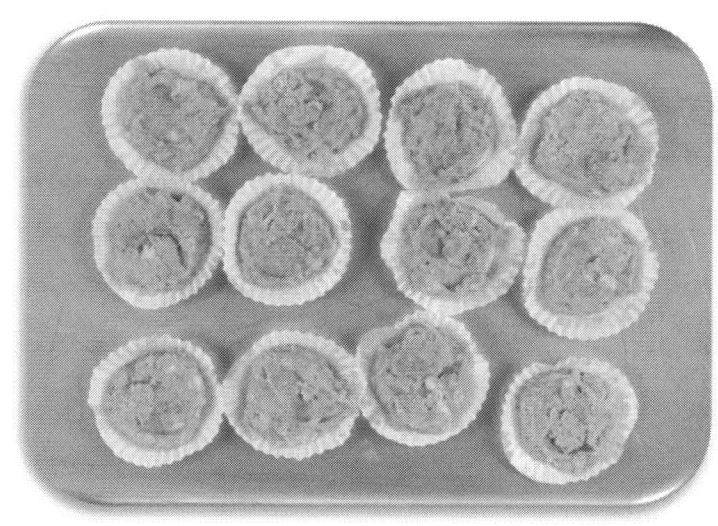

Ingredients:

- ½ cup coconut oil, melted
- ½ cup golden ghee, melted
- 3 Tbsp organic heavy whipping cream
- 1 cup peanut butter, smooth
- 1 avocado, peeled, pitted, chopped
- 1 Tbsp sugar-free vanilla bean sweetener

Instructions:

1. In a blender, process all ingredients until smooth.Place the mixture in silicone candy molds. Freeze for at least 3 hours before serving.

Pecan Fudge

Prep time: 45 minutes

Cooking time: 15 minutes

Servings: 60 pieces

Nutrition facts per serving:

Total carbs – 6 g

Protein – 1 g

Total fat – 3 g

Calories – 59

Ingredients:

- ½ cup butter (cubed) + 1 tsp for greasing
- ½ cup whipping cream
- 1 cup chopped pecans, toasted
- 1 tsp vanilla extract
- 1 cup powdered sweetener of your choice
- 1 cup powdered sweetener

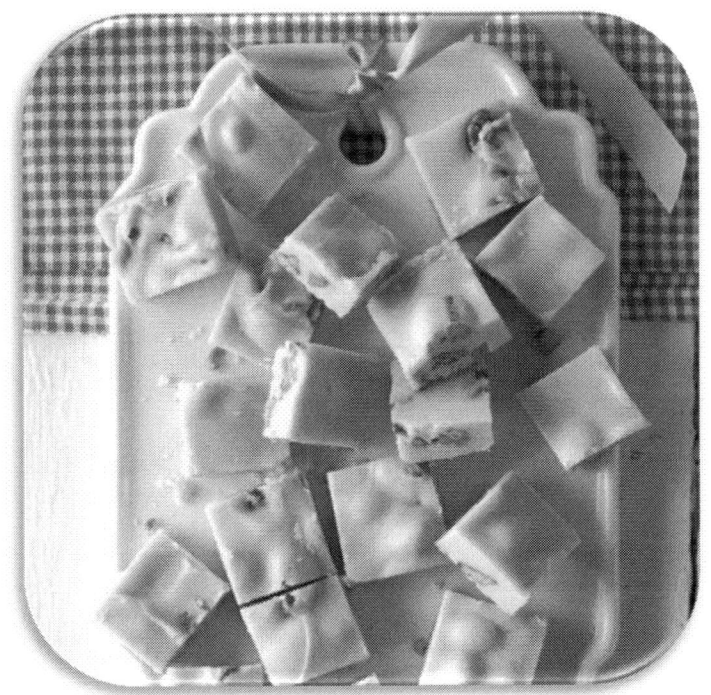

Instructions:

1. In a saucepan heat butter with cream and sweetener of your choice. Bring to a boil constantly stirring. Cook until soft ball stage.
2. Remove from heat and add vanilla.
3. Let cool for about 30 minutes.
4. Beat the fudge with a fork until it begins to thicken. Stir in the powdered sweetener gradually until smooth.
5. Add the nuts and stir.
6. Spread the fudge into a greased baking pan. Cover with foil and cool in the fridge.
7. Remove the foil and cut into squares.

Coconut-Raspberry Fat Bombs

Prep time: 3 hours 15 minutes

Cooking time: 0 minutes

Servings: 12

Nutrients per serving:

Carbohydrates – 3.2 g

Net Carbs – 2.5 g

Fat – 18 g

Protein – 0.3 g

Calories – 169

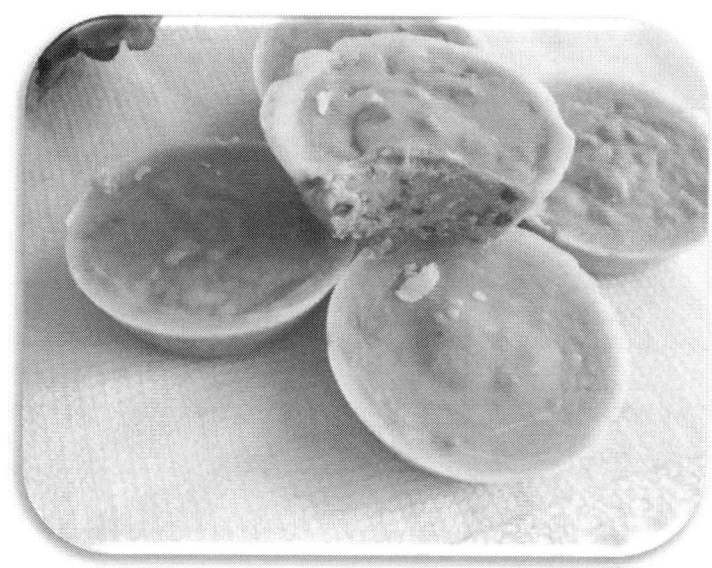

Ingredients:

- ½ cup coconut butter
- ½ cup coconut oil
- ½ cup freeze dried raspberries
- ½ cup unsweetened shredded coconut
- ¼ powdered sugar substitutes such as Swerve or Truvia

Instructions:

1. Line an 8x8 pan with parchment paper.
2. In a food processor, pulse the dried raspberries into a fine powder.
3. In a saucepan over medium heat, combine the coconut butter, coconut oil, coconut, and sweetener. Stir until melted and well combined.
4. Remove pan from heat and stir in raspberry powder.
5. Add mixture into silicone molds and freeze for overnight.
6. Pop fat bombs out of molds and serve.

Chocolate-Coconut Layered Cups

Prep time: 25 minutes

Cooking time: 0 minutes

Servings: 10

Nutrients per serving:

Carbohydrates – 2.7 g

Net Carbs – 0.35 g

Fat – 27.5 g

Protein – 1 g

Calories – 247

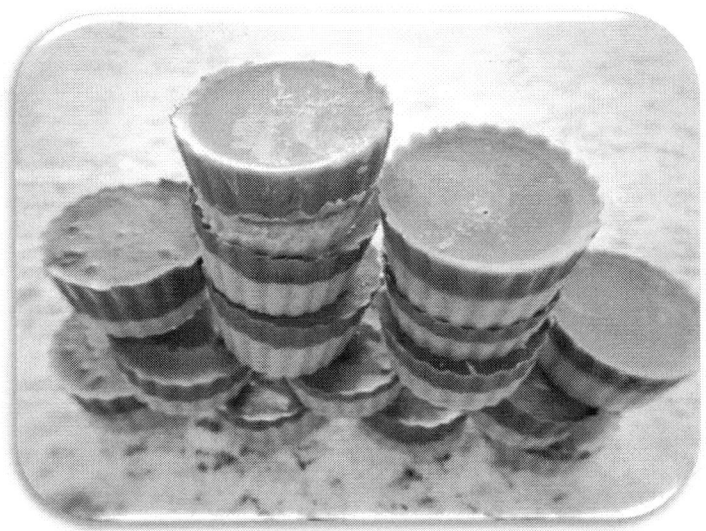

Ingredients:

- ½ cup coconut butter
- ½ cup coconut oil
- ½ cup unsweetened, shredded coconut
- 3 Tbsp powdered sweetener such as Splenda or Truvia
- ½ cup cocoa butter
- 1 oz unsweetened chocolate
- ½ tsp vanilla extract

Instructions:

1. Prepare a mini-muffin pan with 20 mini paper liners.
2. Combine coconut butter and coconut oil in a saucepan over low heat. Stir until smooth, then add the shredded coconut and powdered sweetener until combined.
3. Divide the mixture among muffin cups and freeze until firm, about 30 minutes.
4. Combine cocoa butter and unsweetened chocolate together in double boiler or a bowl set over a pan of simmering water. Stir until melted.
5. Stir in the powdered sweetener, then the cocoa powder and mix until smooth.
6. Remove from heat and add the vanilla extract.
7. Spoon chocolate topping over chilled coconut candies and let set, about 15 minutes. Serve.

Frozen Coffee Hazelnut Coconut

Prep time: 3 hours 15 minutes

Cooking time: 5 minutes

Servings: 12

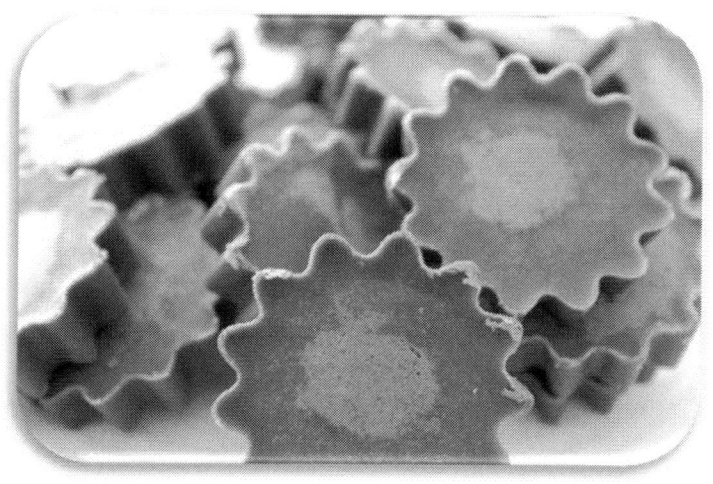

Nutrients per serving:

Carbohydrates – 2 g

Net Carbs – 0.47 g

Fat – 8 g

Protein – 2 g

Calories – 96

Ingredients:

- ¼ cup coconut oil
- ¼ cup almond butter
- 1 tsp instant coffee granules
- 12 drops liquid stevia
- 2 Tbsp cocoa powder
- 12 hazelnuts

Instructions:

1. Combine coconut oil, almond butter, coffee, and stevia in a small saucepan over medium heat, frequently stirring until ingredients have melted. Turn off heat.
2. Add cocoa powder and stir well to combine.
3. Pour mixture into 12 molds of a silicone-bottomed ice cube tray or silicone candy mold tray.
4. Place 1 hazelnut into each filled mold.
5. Freeze until set. Serve from the freezer.

Frozen Orange Creamsicle

Prep time: 3 hours 15 minutes

Cooking time: 0 minutes

Servings: 12

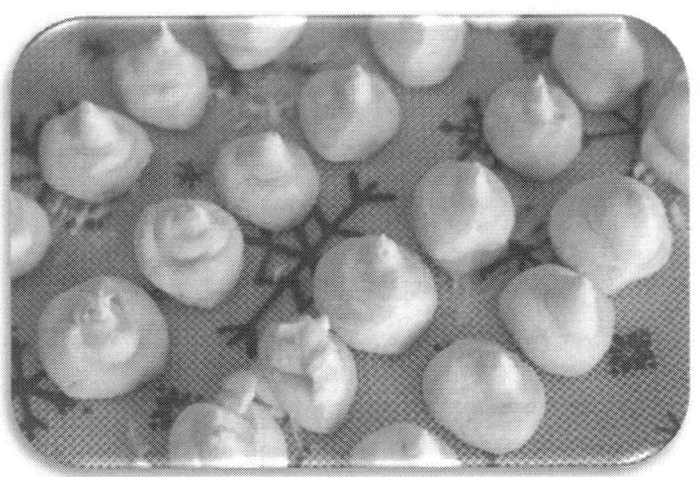

Nutrients per serving:

Carbohydrates – 1 g

Net Carbs – 0.48 g

Fat –8g

Protein – 0 g

Calories – 75

Ingredients:

- ¼cup coconut oil
- ¼ cup heavy whipping cream
- 2 oz cream cheese, softened
- 2 Tbsp orange juice, freshly squeezed
- 1 Tbsp orange zest
- 12 drops liquid stevia

Instructions:

1. Blend all ingredients with an immersion blender, about 30 seconds.
2. Spoon mixture into 12 molds of a silicone candy mold tray.
3. Freeze until set. Serve from the freezer.

Frozen Matcha Cream

Prep time: 3 hours 20 minutes

Cooking time: 0 minutes

Servings: 12

Nutrients per serving:

Carbohydrates – 6 g

Net Carbs – 2 g

Fat –9 g

Protein – 0 g

Calories – 103

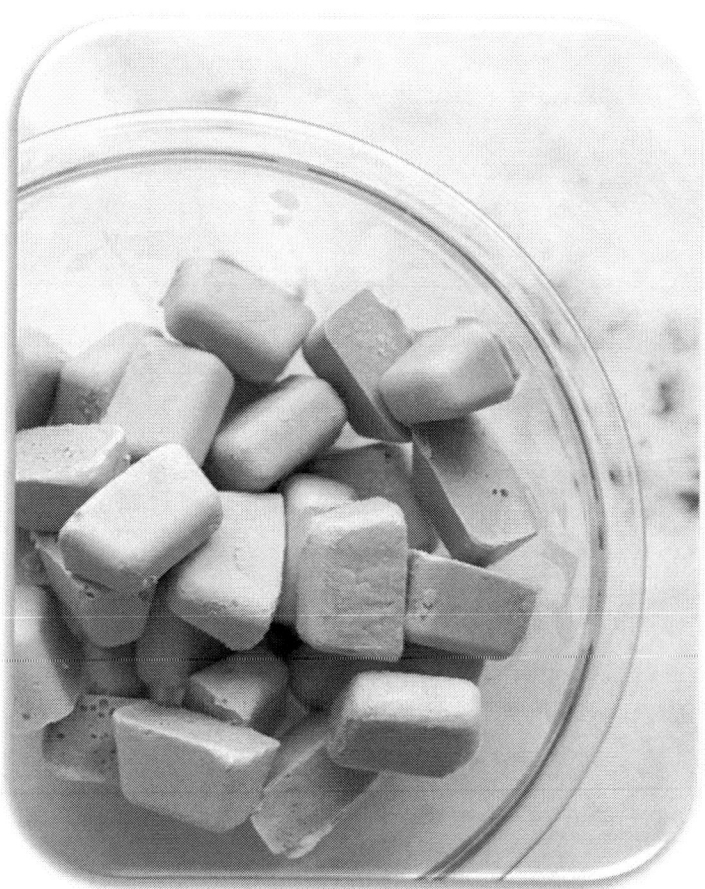

Ingredients:

- 3 oz cocoa butter
- 3 oz coconut cream
- 1 Tbsp coconut oil
- ½ tsp matcha
- 2 Tbsp confectioners Swerve
- 2 drops stevia glycerite
- 1/8 tsp sea salt
- 2 Tbsp matcha

Instructions:

1. In a small double boiler over medium-low heat, melt cocoa butter while stirring slowly.
2. Add coconut cream, coconut oil, ½ tsp matcha, Swerve, stevia, and sea salt. Mix well.
3. Remove from heat and stir for about 10 seconds.
4. Pour into a silicone mold for chocolate or candy in the desired shape. Molds should be about 1" deep and 1½ " wide.
5. Freeze at least 3 hours or overnight. Once frozen, remove shapes from molds then sprinkle with 2 Tbsp matcha to coat tops.

Almond Cookie Popsicles

Prep time: 8 hours 15 minutes

Cooking time: 0 minutes

Servings: 8

Nutrients per serving:

Carbohydrates – 9 g

Net Carbs –4 g

Fat –17 g

Protein – 5 g

Calories – 294

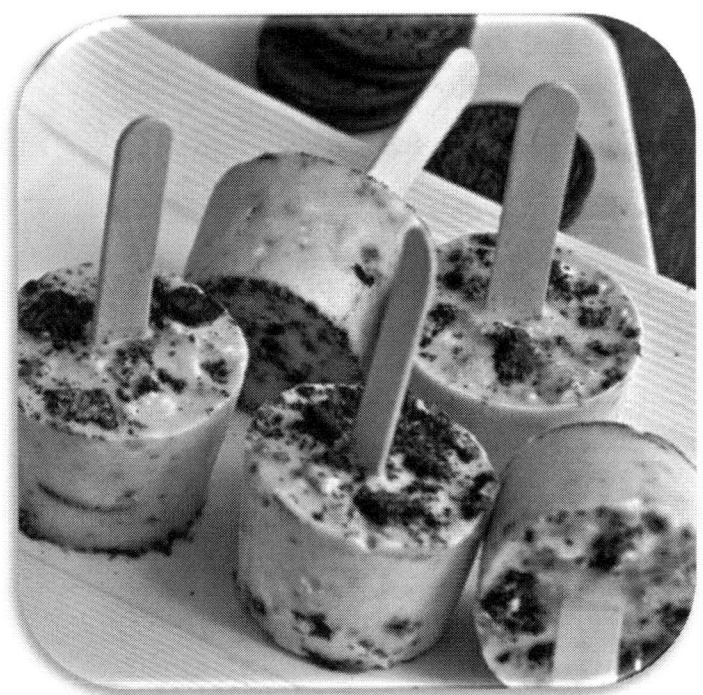

Ingredients:

- 1½ cups coconut cream, chilled
- ½ cup almond butter
- 1 tsp vanilla extract
- ¼ erythritol or granular Swerve

Instructions:

1. Put all ingredients in a blender and process until completely mixed, about 30 seconds
2. Pour mix into 8 popsicle molds, tapping molds to dislodge air bubbles.
3. Freeze at least 8 hours or overnight.

Orange Chocolate Popsicles

Prep time: 8 hours 15 minutes

Cooking time: 0 minutes

Servings: 4

Nutrients per serving:

Carbohydrates – 23 g

Net Carbs –11 g

Fat –15 g

Protein – 4 g

Calories – 237

Ingredients:

- 1 medium avocado
- ½ cup coconut cream
- ½ cup cocoa powder
- 2 Tbsp erythritol or granular Swerve
- 1 tsp orange zest
- 1/8 tsp orange extract
- 1/8 tsp salt

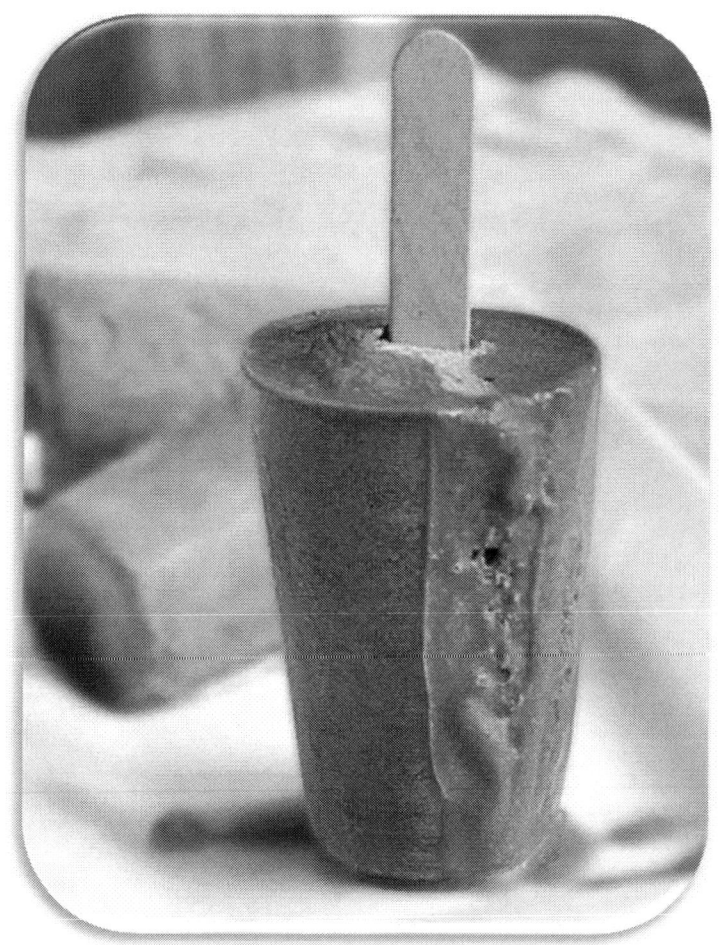

Instructions:

1. Blend all ingredients in a food processor until completely mixed, about 30 seconds.
2. Pour mix into 4 popsicle molds, tapping molds to dislodge air bubbles.
3. Freeze at least 8 hours or overnight.

Mint Chocolate Chip Popsicles

Prep time: 8 hours 20 minutes

Cooking time: 5 minutes

Servings: 8

Nutrients per serving:

Carbohydrates – 10 g

Net Carbs – 6 g

Fat – 16 g

Protein – 2 g

Calories – 304

Ingredients:

- 2 cups coconut milk
- 1 cup fresh mint leaves
- 2 oz unsweetened chocolate chips
- ¼ cup erythritol or granular Swerve

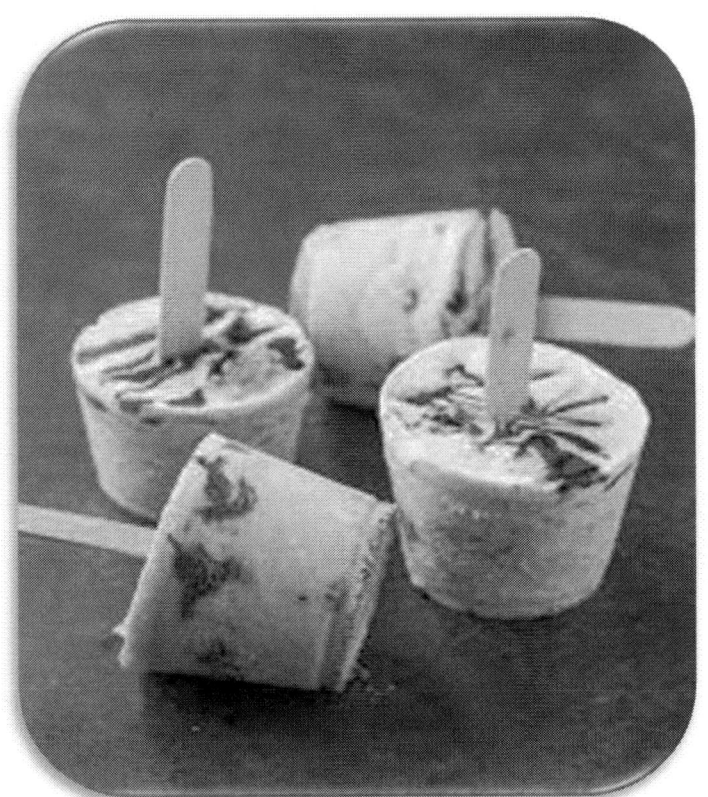

Instructions:

1. Combine coconut milk and mint in a medium saucepan over medium heat.
2. Simmer until bubbles start appearing, about 5 minutes. Remove from heat and ssset aside for 20 minutes.
3. Strain through a fine-mesh sieve into a bowl.
4. Add chocolate and sweetener and stir well.
5. Pour mix into 8 popsicle molds, tapping molds to dislodge air bubbles.
6. Freeze at least 8 hours or overnight.

Hazelnut Cappuccino Popsicles

Prep time: 8 hours 15 minutes

Cooking time: 1 minute

Servings: 8

Nutrients per serving:

Carbohydrates – 8 g

Net Carbs – 6 g

Fat – 15 g

Protein – 2 g

Calories – 148

Ingredients:

- 1 cup brewed espresso or strong coffee
- 1 cup heavy whipping cream
- 1/8 tsp hazelnut flavor
- ¼ cup erythritol or granular Swerve

Instructions:

1. Place all ingredients except hazelnuts in a blender and blend until completely mixed, about 30 seconds.

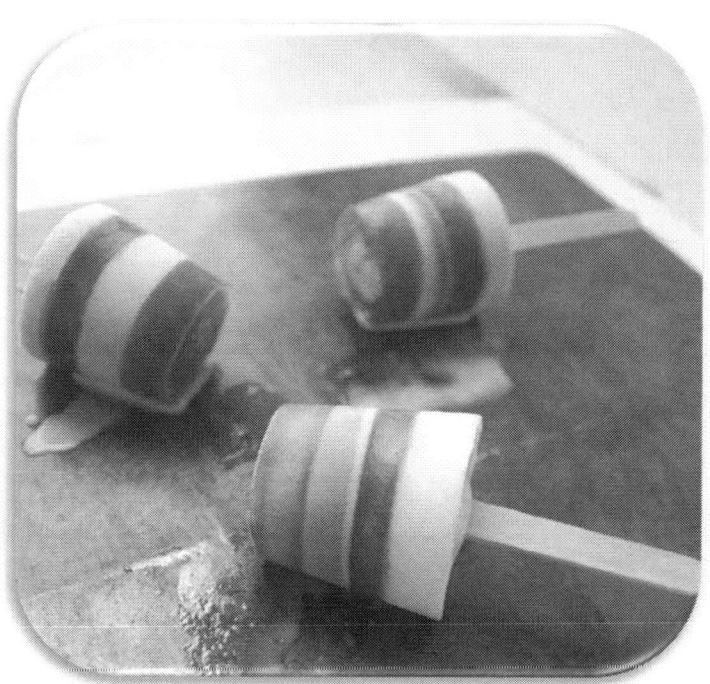

2. Pour mix into 8 popsicle molds, tapping molds to dislodge air bubbles. 3. Freeze at least 8 hours or overnight.
3. In a nonstick pan over medium heat, toast crumbled hazelnuts for 1 minute, stirring constantly.
4. Remove popsicles from molds. If popsicles are hard to remove from containers, run molds under hot water briefly and popsicles will come loose.

Ginger Cream Popsicles

Prep time: 8 hours 10 minutes

Cooking time: 0 minutes

Servings: 8

Nutrients per serving:

Carbohydrates – 14 g

Net Carbs – 9 g

Fat –15 g

Protein – 1 g

Calories – 295

Ingredients:

- 2 cups coconut milk chilled
- 2 Tbsp coconut oil
- 1 tsp ground ginger
- ¼ cup erythritol or granular Swerve

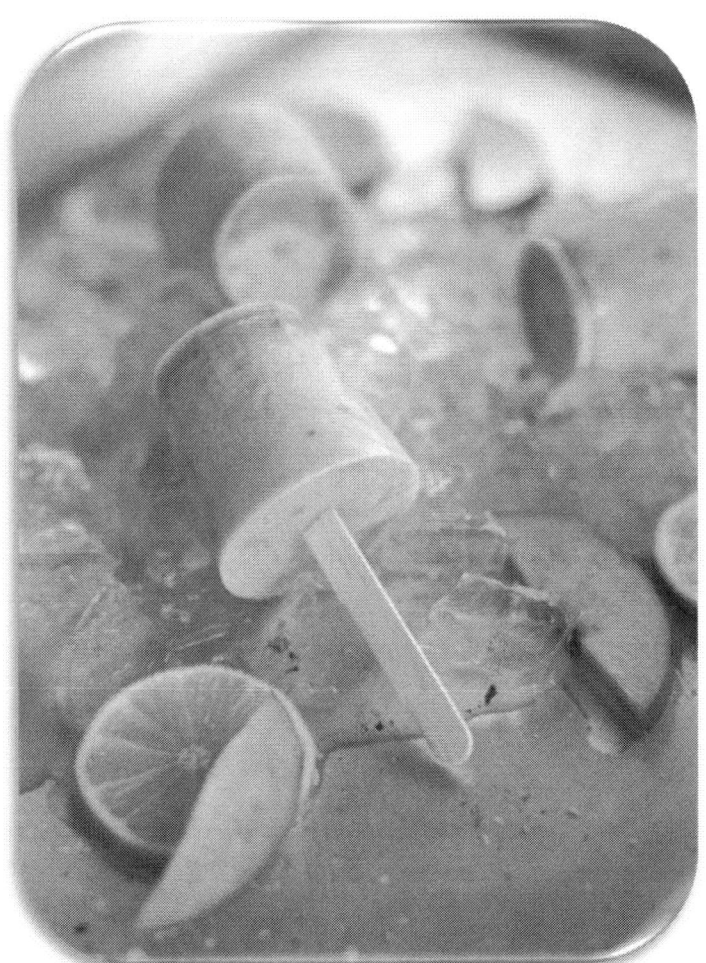

Instructions:

1. Put all ingredients in a blender and blend until completely mixed, about 30 seconds.
2. Pour mix into 8 popsicle molds, tapping molds to dislodge air bubbles.
3. Freeze at least 8 hours or overnight.

CONCLUSION

Thank you for reading this book and having the patience to try the recipes.

I do hope that you gain as much enjoyment reading and experimenting with the meals as I have had writing this book.

If you would like to leave a comment, you can do it at the Order section->Digital orders, in your amazon account.

Stay safe and healthy!

Recipe Index

Conversion Tables

VALUE EQUIVALENTS (LIQUID)

US STANDARD	US STANDARD (OUNCES)	METRIC (VOLUME)
2 tablespoons	1 fl. oz.	30 mL
¼ cup	2 fl. oz.	60 mL
½ cup	4 fl. oz.	120 mL
1 cup	8 fl. oz.	240mL
1 ½ cup	12 fl. oz.	355 mL
2 cups or 1 pint	16 fl. oz.	`475 mL
4 cups or 1 quart	32 fl. oz.	1 L
1 gallon	128 fl. oz.	4 L

OVEN TEMPERATURES

FAHRENHEIT(F)	CELSIUS(C) APPROXIMATE
250 °F	120 °C
300 °F	150 °C
325 °F	165 °C
350 °F	180 °C
375 °F	190°C
400 °F	200 °C
425 °F	220 °C
450 °F	230 °C

VALUE EQUIVALENTS (LIQUID)

US STANDARD	METRIC (APPROXIMATE)
$\frac{1}{8}$ teaspoon	0.5 mL
¼ teaspoon	1 mL
½ teaspoon	2 mL
$\frac{2}{3}$ teaspoon	4 mL
1 teaspoon	5 mL
1 tablespoon	15 mL
¼ cup	59 mL
$\frac{1}{3}$ cup	79 mL
½ cup	118 mL
$\frac{2}{3}$ cup	156 mL
¾ cup	177 mL
1 cup	235 mL
2 cups or 1 pint	475 mL
3 cups	700 mL
4 cups or 1 quart	1 L
½ gallon	2 L
1 gallon	4 L

WEIGHT EQUIVALENTS

US STANDARD	METRIC (APPROXIMATE)
½ ounce	15 g
1 ounces	30 g
2 ounces	60 g
4 ounces	115 g
8 ounces	225 g
12 ounces	340 g
16 ounce or 1 pound	455 g

Other Books by Adele Baker

Adele Baker's page on Amazon https://goo.gl/szoZSY

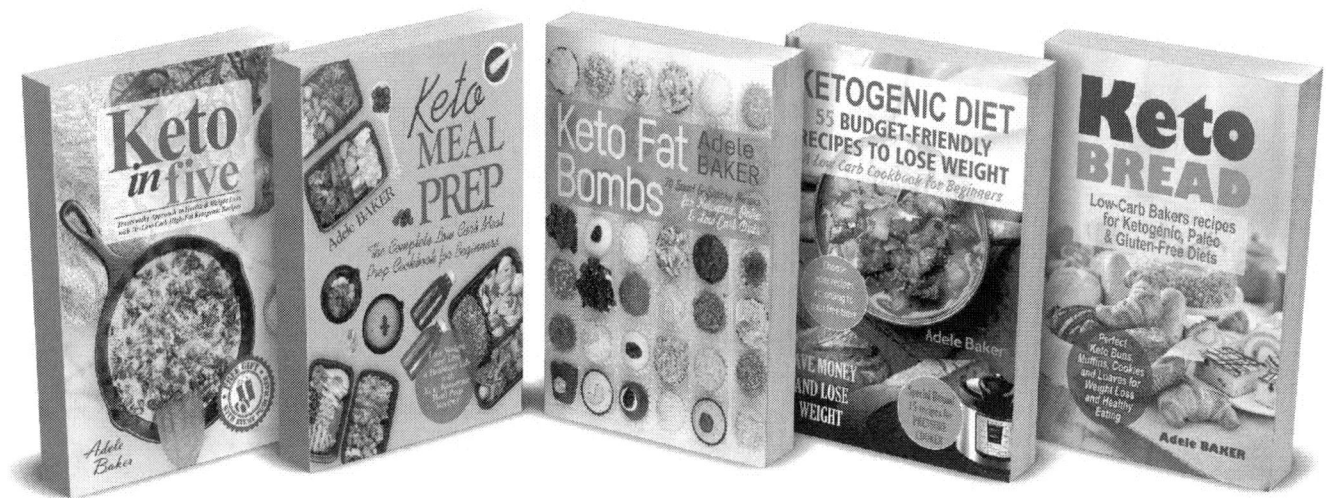

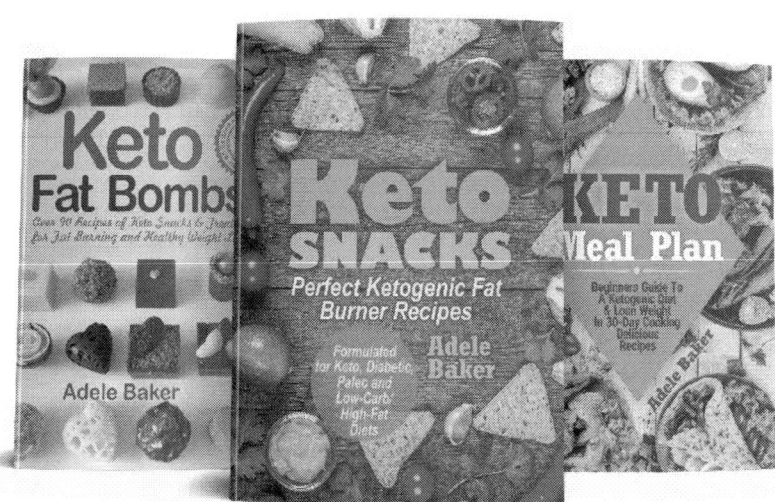

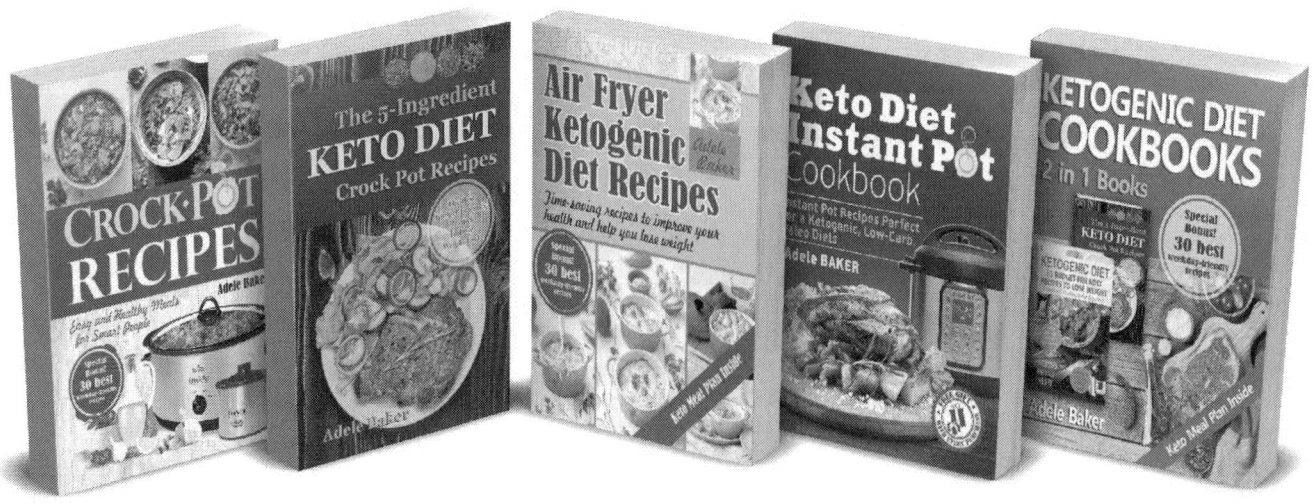

Made in the USA
Lexington, KY
09 March 2019